a LANGE medica

MW00964046

CURRENT

ESSENTIALS
of SURGERY

Gerard M. Doherty, MD
N.W. Thompson Professor of Surgery
Section Head, General Surgery
University of Michigan
Ann Arbor

Lange Medical Books/McGraw-Hill
Medical Publishing Division

New York   Chicago   San Francisco   Lisbon   London   Madrid   Mexico City
Milan   New Delhi   San Juan   Seoul   Singapore   Sydney   Toronto

Current Essentials of Surgery

2   3   4   5   6   7   8   9   0   DOCDOC   0   9   8   7   6   5

ISBN: 0-07-142314-1
ISSN: 1553-8370

This book was set in Adobe Garamond by International Typesetting and Composition.
The editors were Marc Strauss, Harriet Lebowitz, and Peter J. Boyle.
The production supervisor was Catherine Saggese.
The art manager was Charissa Baker.
The text was designed by Eve Siegel.
The index was prepared by Kathrin Unger.
R.R. Donnelly was printer and binder.

This book is printed on acid-free paper.

Contents

Contributors

Gorav Ailawadi, MD
Department of Surgery
University of Michigan
Ann Arbor
Noncardiac Thoracic Surgery; Adult Cardiac Surgery; Congenital Cardiac Surgery; Arteries; Veins & Lymphatics

Charles E. Binkley, MD
Department of Surgery
University of Michigan
Ann Arbor
Esophagus & Diaphragm; Stomach & Duodenum; Pancreas; Spleen; Small Intestine

Derek A. DuBay, MD
Department of Surgery
University of Michigan
Ann Arbor
Acute Abdomen; Peritoneal Cavity; Hernias; Sarcoma, Lymphoma, & Melanoma

Theodore R. Lin, MD
Department of Surgery
University of Michigan
Ann Arbor
Surgical Infections; Colon; Anorectum

John W. McGillicuddy, MD
Department of Surgery
University of Michigan
Ann Arbor
Fluids & Electrolytes; Shock & Acute Pulmonary Failure; Trauma; Burns & Thermal Injury

Brian D. Saunders, MD
Department of Surgery
University of Michigan
Ann Arbor
Head & Neck; Thyroid & Parathyroid; Breast; Adrenals

Theodore H. Welling III, MD
Department of Surgery
University of Michigan
Ann Arbor
Liver & Portal Venous System; Biliary Tract; Pediatric Surgery

Preface

Current Essentials of Surgery, organized by body system and disease, is designed to provide rapid access to important information regarding general surgery problems. This book was compiled by a select group of residents from the General Surgery training program at the University of Michigan and covers the information we expect residents and medical students, in particular, to know. The individual topics included in each body system chapter are the important diseases that must be considered in a general surgery differential diagnosis. Concisely presented within each disease topic are the Essentials of the Diagnosis, the Differential Diagnosis to consider for that disorder, the Treatment of the condition, and relevant Reference material. For further emphasis, there is also a Clinical Pearl that highlights an important teaching point for each entry.

We hope that *Current Essentials of Surgery* will be a useful resource for medical students and junior residents in surgery. It provides the necessary background material from which to build a solid fund of knowledge in the field of surgery.

Gerard M. Doherty, MD
Ann Arbor, Michigan

Section I

Burn, Trauma & Critical Care

Chapters

1

Fluids & Electrolytes

Acidosis, Metabolic

- ■ Essentials of Diagnosis
  - Decreased serum pH (<7.35)
  - Decreased serum HCO_3
  - Causes include diarrhea, diuretics, renal tubular disease, ureterosigmoidostomy, lactic acidosis, diabetic ketoacidosis, uremia
  - Diagnostic tests include arterial blood gas (ABG) measurements
  - Calculate anion gap: $Na - (Cl + HCO_3)$
  - Anion gap >15: H^+ excess, lactic acidosis, diabetic ketoacidosis, uremia, methanol ingestion, salicylate intoxication, ethylene glycol ingestion
  - Anion gap <15: HCO_3 loss, diarrhea, renal tubular disease, ureterosigmoidostomy, acetazolamide, NH_4 Cl administration

- ■ Differential Diagnosis
  - Differentiate between anion gap or hyperchloremic causes

- ■ Treatment
  - Conservative HCO_3 administration
  - Estimate need by multiplying base deficit by one half total body water

- ■ Pearls

Gap acidosis = SLUMPED: salicylates, lactate, uremia, methanol, paraldehyde, ethylene glycol, diabetes.

Non-gap acidosis = 2 renal (renal tubular acidosis, renal failure), 2 gastrointestinal (enterocutaneous fistula, urine diversion to gastrointestinal tract), and 2 drugs (ammonium chloride, acetazolamide).

Reference

Adrogue HJ et al: Management of life-threatening acid-base disorders [two parts]. N Engl J Med 1998;338:26, 107.

Acidosis, Respiratory

- **Essentials of Diagnosis**
  - Inadequate ventilation
  - Carbon dioxide accumulation
  - Somnolence
  - Decreased serum pH (<7.35)
  - Increased P_{CO_2}
  - Causes include acute airway obstruction, aspiration, respiratory arrest, pulmonary infections, pulmonary edema, chronic respiratory failure

- **Differential Diagnosis**
  - Causes may be neurologic, mechanical, or rarely from diffusion abnormality
  - May be acute or chronic

- **Treatment**
  - Restore adequate ventilation
  - Intubate if necessary
  - Chronic or rapid correction may lead to severe metabolic alkalosis (post-hypercapnic metabolic alkalosis)
  - Perform serial ABG measurements

- **Pearl**

Ensure adequate ventilation.

Reference

Adrogue HJ et al: Management of life-threatening acid-base disorders [two parts]. N Engl J Med 1998;338:26, 107.

Alkalosis, Metabolic

- **Essentials of Diagnosis**
  - Elevated serum pH (>7.45)
  - Increased serum HCO_3
  - Most common acid-base disturbance in surgical patients
  - Pathogenesis involves loss of H^+ via nasogastric suction, volume depletion, and hypokalemia
  - Paradoxical aciduria
  - Hypokalemia
  - Diagnostic tests include serum electrolytes, ABG measurement, urine electrolytes, urine pH

- **Differential Diagnosis**
  - May be mixed, most commonly with respiratory acidosis, but ventilatory compensation is limited
  - Usually marked volume depletion

- **Treatment**
  - Fluid resuscitation (usually with normal saline)
  - Potassium repletion as KCl
  - Monitor treatment with serial ABG measurements

- **Pearl**

Correct volume; kidneys will correct pH.

Reference

Adrogue HJ et al: Management of life-threatening acid-base disorders [two parts]. N Engl J Med 1998;338:26, 107.

Alkalosis, Respiratory

- **Essentials of Diagnosis**
  - Acute hyperventilation lowers $PaCO_2$ without concomitant changes in plasma bicarbonate concentration
  - Chronic respiratory alkalosis occurs in pulmonary and liver disease
  - May be an early sign of sepsis
  - Paresthesias
  - Carpopedal spasm
  - Positive Chvostek sign

- **Differential Diagnosis**
  - Electrolyte pattern of chronic respiratory alkalosis is the same as in hyperchloremic acidosis; they can be distinguished only by ABG pH measurement
  - May be a sign of sepsis, pulmonary embolus, or other stress

- **Treatment**
  - Chronic respiratory alkalosis does not generally require treatment
  - Treatment of chronic respiratory alkalosis may lead to metabolic acidosis and hyperchloremia

- **Pearl**

Respiratory alkalosis is usually a symptom; find the underlying cause.

Reference

Adrogue HJ et al: Management of life-threatening acid-base disorders [two parts]. N Engl J Med 1998;338:26, 107.

Dehydration (Volume & Electrolyte Depletion)

- **Essentials of Diagnosis**
  - Water deficit without solute deficit
  - Water deficit can be estimated from serum Na concentration: water deficit = [(140 − serum Na) × total body water]/140
  - Occurs in patients unable to regulate water intake
  - Rare in surgical patients
  - Insensible water loss from fever
  - Tube feedings with inadequate water content
  - Diabetes insipidus
  - Concentrated urine
  - Central nervous system depression
  - Lethargy
  - Coma
  - Muscle rigidity
  - Tremors
  - Spasticity
  - Seizures
  - Hypernatremia
  - Low urine Na despite hypernatremia

- **Differential Diagnosis**
  - Pure water deficit occurs in people unable to regulate their own intake and in diabetes insipidus
  - Water deficit is usually accompanied by solute (Na^+) deficit

- **Treatment**
  - Replace enough water to return serum Na concentration to normal
  - Treat patient with D5W unless hypotension has developed, in which case use hypotonic saline
  - Monitor serum Na

- **Pearl**

Correct intravascular volume first, then slowly replenish water deficit.

Reference

Palevsky PM et al: Hypernatremia in hospitalized patients. Ann Intern Med 1996;124:197.

Hypercalcemia

- **Essentials of Diagnosis**
  - Elevated serum calcium
  - Fatigability
  - Muscle weakness
  - Depression
  - Anorexia
  - Nausea
  - Constipation
  - Polyuria
  - Polydipsia
  - Metastatic calcification
  - Coma
  - Excess parathyroid hormone (PTH)
  - Perform physical examination

- **Differential Diagnosis**
  - Hyperparathyroidism
  - Cancer with bone metastases
  - Ectopic PTH production
  - Vitamin D intoxication
  - Hyperthyroidism
  - Milk-alkali syndrome
  - Prolonged immobilization
  - Thiazide diuretics
  - Addison disease

- **Treatment**
  - If severe (>14.5 mg/dL), intravenous (IV) isotonic saline should be given
  - Furosemide
  - IV sodium sulfate
  - Plicamycin is useful to treat those with metastatic cancer
  - Corticosteroids for sarcoidosis, vitamin D intoxication, and Addison disease
  - Calcitonin can be useful for patients with impaired renal or cardiac function who might not tolerate forced diuresis

- **Pearl**

Hyperparathyroidism is the only cause of hypercalcemia with PTH >15% above normal.

Reference

Bilezikian JP: Management of acute hypercalcemia. N Engl J Med 1992;326:1196.

Hyperkalemia

- Essentials of Diagnosis
  - Elevated serum potassium
  - Causes include severe trauma, burns, crush injuries, renal insufficiency, marked catabolism, Addison disease

- Differential Diagnosis
  - Addison disease
  - Rule out hemolysis, leukocytosis, thrombocytosis ($>1,000,000/\mu L$), abnormalities of acid-base status (acidosis), tissue necrosis, acute renal failure, excessive KCl with renal dysfunction

- Treatment
  - IV 100 mL D50 with 20 U regular insulin
  - IV $NaHCO_3$
  - IV calcium
  - Sodium polystyrene sulfonate orally or by enema (40–80 g/d)
  - Hemodialysis
  - β-Agonists (inhaled)

- Pearl

Do not give IV potassium until urine production is assured.

Reference

Greenberg A: Hyperkalemia: Treatment options. Semin Nephrol 1998;18:46.

Hypermagnesemia

- **Essentials of Diagnosis**
  - Renal insufficiency
  - Elevated serum magnesium
  - Usually occurs in patients with renal disease
  - Rare in surgical patients
  - Lethargy
  - Weakness
  - Widened QRS complex
  - Depressed ST segment
  - Peaked T waves

- **Differential Diagnosis**
  - When serum level reaches 6 mEq/L, deep tendon reflexes are lost
  - Levels >10 mEq/L can lead to somnolence, coma, and death

- **Treatment**
  - IV isotonic saline to increase renal excretion
  - Slow IV infusion of calcium
  - Dialysis may be necessary
  - Monitor treatment with electrocardiogram and serum magnesium levels

- **Pearl**

Eliminate magnesium-containing antacids in patients with renal failure.

Reference

Whang R: Clinical disorders of magnesium metabolism. Compr Ther 1997;23:168.

Hypernatremia

- **Essentials of Diagnosis**
  - High serum sodium
  - Caused by either a loss of water or a gain of hypertonic saline
  - Typically accompanies dehydration or water loss in perioperative or post-trauma patients

- **Differential Diagnosis**
  - Pure water loss: unreplaced insensible water losses, neurogenic diabetes insipidus, congenital diabetes insipidus, acquired nephrogenic diabetes insipidus
  - Hypertonic sodium gain: hypertonic sodium bicarbonate infusion, hypertonic feeding solution, sodium chloride ingestion, sea water ingestion or drowning, hypertonic sodium chloride infusion, primary hyperaldosteronism, Cushing syndrome
  - Must determine intravascular volume status to guide resuscitation

- **Treatment**
  - Water replacement, sodium restriction, or both
  - Change serum sodium no more than 1–2 mEq/L/h; more rapid changes risk iatrogenic cerebral edema
  - Monitor treatment with serum electrolytes

- **Pearl**

Change serum sodium slowly.

Reference

Adrogue HJ, Madias NE: Hypernatremia. N Engl J Med 2000;342:1493.

Hyperphosphatemia

- **Essentials of Diagnosis**
  - Elevated serum phosphorus
  - Renal insufficiency
  - Trauma
  - Marked tissue catabolism
  - Excess intake (rarely)
  - Usually asymptomatic

- **Differential Diagnosis**
  - In perioperative or post-trauma setting, almost always associated with renal insufficiency, even when other factors are also present

- **Treatment**
  - Diuresis
  - Phosphate binding materials
  - Dialysis
  - Monitor treatment with serum electrolytes

- **Pearl**

Monitor phosphorus when resuming nutrition.

Reference

Klahr S et al: Acute renal failure. N Engl J Med 1998;338:671.

Hypocalcemia

- ■ Essentials of Diagnosis
  - Depressed serum calcium
  - Post thyroidectomy or parathyroidectomy
  - Hyperactive deep tendon reflexes
  - Chvostek sign
  - Muscle or abdominal cramps
  - Carpopedal spasm
  - Convulsions

- ■ Differential Diagnosis
  - Hypoparathyroidism
  - Hypomagnesemia
  - Severe pancreatitis
  - Renal failure
  - Severe trauma
  - Crush injuries
  - Necrotizing fasciitis

- ■ Treatment
  - Treat alkalosis if present
  - Acute treatment: calcium gluconate 6 g in 500 mL D5W; infuse at 1 mL/kg/h; monitor serum calcium and adjust infusion as necessary
  - Long-term treatment: vitamin D, oral calcium, phosphate binders
  - Monitor treatment with serum calcium; ionized calcium

- ■ Pearl

Use IV calcium gluconate infusion rather than bolus to avoid a roller-coaster effect.

Reference

Lebowitz MR et al: Hypocalcemia. Semin Nephrol 1992;12:146.

Hypokalemia

- ### Essentials of Diagnosis
  - Depressed serum potassium
  - Decreased muscle contractility
  - Paralysis
  - Causes include alcoholism, elderly patients, prolonged NPO status
  - Diagnostic tests include serum electrolytes including magnesium, ABG (pH) measurement, urine potassium losses (<30 mEq/d total body deficit; >30 mEq/d renal wasting)

- ### Differential Diagnosis
  - Laboratory error or difficulty with phlebotomy; blood drawn from above an IV infusion can give spurious results with very low potassium
  - Rule out hypomagnesemia

- ### Treatment
  - Correct underlying problem
  - Replace potassium
  - Replace magnesium if necessary
  - Correct alkalosis if present
  - Give KCl orally if possible, or give 20–30 mEq/h IV by central vein or 10 mEq/h by peripheral vein
  - Administer $MgSO_4$

- ### Pearl

For a postoperative potassium <2.8, bring the defibrillator to the bedside.

References

Kruse JA et al: Rapid correction of hypokalemia using concentrated intravenous potassium chloride infusions. Arch Intern Med 1990;150:613.

Whang R et al: Refractory potassium repletion: A consequence of magnesium deficiency. Arch Intern Med 1992;152:40.

Hypomagnesemia

- **Essentials of Diagnosis**
  - Low serum magnesium
  - Hyperactive deep tendon reflexes
  - Positive Chvostek sign
  - Tremors
  - Delirium
  - Convulsions

- **Differential Diagnosis**
  - Depends on clinical suspicion and serum levels
  - Occurs with poor dietary intake, intestinal malabsorption, or excessive losses from the gut
  - Can also be caused by excessive urine losses, chronic alcohol abuse, hyperaldosteronism, and hypercalcemia
  - Occasionally, develops in acute pancreatitis, diabetic acidosis, burn victims, or with prolonged administration of total parenteral nutrition

- **Treatment**
  - Administer supplemental magnesium
  - Replace orally for mild to moderate hypomagnesemia
  - For severe deficit, give IV magnesium sulfate

- **Pearl**

Be very careful with magnesium in patients with renal failure.

Reference

Kelepouris E et al: Hypomagnesemia: Renal magnesium handling. Semin Nephrol 1998;18:58.

Hyponatremia

- ■ Essentials of Diagnosis
  - Low serum sodium
  - Mental obtundation (sodium <120 mEq/L)
  - Occurs in postoperative patients; premenopausal women after surgery

- ■ Differential Diagnosis
  - Must determine intravascular volume status to guide resuscitation

- ■ Treatment
  - Replace sodium
  - Give hypertonic sodium when condition is severe
  - Raise serum sodium no more than 1–2 mEq/L/h

- ■ Pearl

Change serum sodium slowly.

Reference

Adrogue HJ et al: Hyponatremia. N Engl J Med 2000;342:1581.

Hypophosphatemia

- ■ Essentials of Diagnosis
  - • Decreased serum phosphorus
  - • Lassitude, weakness, and fatigue may develop with levels <1 mg/dL
  - • Severe neuromuscular manifestations can include convulsions and death
  - • Impaired cardiac contractility and rhabdomyolysis with ongoing severe hypophosphatemia
  - • Causes include poor dietary intake (especially in alcoholics), hyperparathyroidism, phosphate-binding antacid administration, refeeding with total parenteral nutrition with insufficient phosphate supplementation

- ■ Differential Diagnosis
  - • In perioperative or post-trauma setting, almost always associated with poor nutrition

- ■ Treatment
  - • Replace phosphate
  - • Give nutritional support
  - • Monitor treatment with serum electrolytes

- ■ Pearl

Monitor phosphorus when resuming nutrition.

Reference

Subramainan R, Khardori R: Severe hypophosphatemia. Pathophysiologic implications, clinical presentations and treatment. Medicine 2000;79:1.

Renal Failure

- ### Essentials of Diagnosis
  - Oliguric (urinary output <400 mL/d) and nonoliguric types
  - Mortality in surgical intensive care unit of 50–90%
  - Causes of parenchymal disease include acute tubular necrosis, pigment nephropathy, nephrotoxic agents, acute rejection after transplantation, prerenal and postrenal causes
  - Laboratory findings include elevated creatinine, hyperkalemia, hyperphosphatemia, elevated blood urea nitrogen, fractional excretion of sodium >3%

- ### Differential Diagnosis
  - Rule out renal artery or vein thrombosis
  - Rule out ureter obstruction or leak

- ### Treatment
  - Medications: optimize cardiac output; perform diuresis and renal replacement therapy (intermittent hemodialysis, continuous venovenous hemofiltration and dialysis if hemodynamically unstable); give adequate nutrition; treat underlying disease; give pulse corticosteroids or OKT3 for acute allograft rejection
  - Prognosis: 50–90% of patients die (highest if oliguric); 90% recover renal function if they survive the underlying inciting illness (recovery unlikely if >6 weeks after resolution of illness)
  - Prevention: Avoid nephrotoxic agents and maintain organ perfusion in the critically ill; ensure adequate immunosuppression and compliance after renal transplantation

- ### Pearl
  Always check prerenal, renal, and postrenal causes.

Reference

Brennan DC: Special medical problems in surgical patients. In Way LW, Doherty GM (editors): Current Surgical Diagnosis & Treatment, 11th ed. McGraw-Hill, 2003.

Volume Overload

- **Essentials of Diagnosis**
  - Volume overload
  - Jugular venous distention
  - Tachypnea
  - Increased body weight
  - Elevated central pressures
  - Causes include postoperative patients, heart failure, liver disease, renal failure, hypoalbuminuria, head injury (syndrome of inappropriate antidiuretic hormone [SIADH]), burns (SIADH), cancer (SIADH)

- **Differential Diagnosis**
  - May be concurrent with myocardial failure or ischemia
  - Examination should include cardiac evaluation

- **Treatment**
  - Sodium restriction
  - Water restriction if low sodium
  - Diuretics if severe
  - Diuretics for SIADH
  - IV isotonic saline to match urinary output (SIADH)

- **Pearl**

Be careful not to overcorrect; it is easier to treat pulmonary edema than death.

Reference

Chang MC et al: Redefining cardiovascular performance during resuscitation: Ventricular stroke work, power, and the pressure-volume diagram. J Trauma 1998;45:470.

2

Shock & Acute Pulmonary Failure

Acute Respiratory Distress Syndrome (ARDS)

- **Essentials of Diagnosis**
  - Hypoxemia
  - Hypercarbia
  - Pulmonary edema (pulmonary capillary wedge pressure <18 mm Hg)
  - Absence of other causes
  - Often follows shock, trauma, or sepsis

- **Differential Diagnosis**
  - ARDS typically develops 24 hours after resuscitation from the initial insult
  - Diagnosis may be complicated by other potential causes of hypoxemia

- **Treatment**
  - Ventilator management (positive end-expiratory pressure, inspiratory reserve volume)
  - Diuresis
  - Treatment of inciting cause
  - Transfusion
  - Proning
  - Invasive monitoring (pulmonary artery catheter)
  - Serial arterial blood gas (ABG) measurements
  - Prognosis: determined by etiology

- **Pearl**

Treat underlying sepsis.

Reference

Bulger EM et al: Current clinical options for the treatment and management of acute respiratory distress syndrome. J Trauma 2000;48:562.

Aspiration

- **Essentials of Diagnosis**
  - Aspiration of gastric contents; hypoxemia
  - Occurs in patients unable to protect the airway, after trauma, in anesthetized patients, or in obtunded patients
  - Vomiting
  - Shortness of breath
  - Gastric contents in airway on bronchoscopy
  - Localized infiltrate on chest film
  - Diagnostic tests include ABG measurements, bronchoscopy

- **Differential Diagnosis**
  - May occur in settings with other causes of hypoxemia (acute respiratory distress syndrome, sepsis, trauma)
  - Patient often has altered level of consciousness

- **Treatment**
  - Pulmonary hygiene
  - Supplemental oxygen
  - Intubation and mechanical ventilation
  - Bronchoscopy
  - Complications include pneumonitis, pneumonia
  - Prognosis: determined by patient's overall health
  - Prevention: aspiration precautions; avoid oversedation

- **Pearl**

Corticosteroid therapy is not helpful.

Reference

Bulger EM et al: Current clinical options for the treatment and management of acute respiratory distress syndrome. J Trauma 2000;48:562.

Atelectasis

- **Essentials of Diagnosis**
  - Localized collapse of alveoli
  - Hypoxemia
  - Bronchial breath sounds over dependent portions of lungs
  - Parenchymal collapse on chest film
  - Small lung volumes on chest film
  - Causes include prolonged immobilization, splinting, prolonged shallow respirations

- **Differential Diagnosis**
  - Frequently occurs within 48 hours postoperatively
  - Fever is often unaccompanied by other findings
  - Differential diagnosis includes other causes of postoperative fever (wound, pulmonary or urinary sepsis, deep vein thrombosis, drugs)

- **Treatment**
  - Encourage deep breathing, ambulation, coughing
  - Perform bronchoscopy, mechanical ventilation, diuresis if appropriate
  - Complications include pneumonia
  - Prognosis is excellent

- **Pearl**

Keep patients upright as much as possible to expand respiratory excursions.

Reference

Celi BR et al: A controlled trial of intermittent positive pressure breathing, incentive spirometry, and deep breathing exercises in preventing pulmonary complications after abdominal surgery. Am Rev Respir Dis 1984;130:12.

Cardiac Compressive Shock

- **Essentials of Diagnosis**
  - Inadequate perfusion
  - Compression of the heart or great veins
  - Pericardial tamponade
  - Tension pneumothorax
  - Abdominal compartment syndrome
  - Diaphragmatic rupture with abdominal viscera in chest
  - Distended neck veins
  - Postural hypotension
  - Oliguria
  - Sweating
  - Mental status changes
  - Paradoxic pulse: a fall of >10 mm Hg with inspiration supports the diagnosis
  - Equalization of heart chamber pressures with pulmonary artery catheter placement

- **Differential Diagnosis**
  - Mechanism of injury often raises suspicion
  - Pericardial tamponade
  - Tension pneumothorax
  - Abdominal compartment syndrome
  - Diaphragmatic rupture with abdominal viscera in chest

- **Treatment**
  - Fluid infusion can bring transient improvement
  - Definitive treatment must correct the mechanical abnormality

- **Pearl**

Hypotension and distended neck veins can be a surgical emergency.

Reference

Asensio JA et al: Penetrating cardiac injuries: A prospective study of variables predicting outcomes. J Am Coll Surg 1998;186:24.

Cardiogenic Shock

- ■ Essentials of Diagnosis
  - • Inadequate tissue perfusion due to heart pump failure

- ■ Differential Diagnosis
  - • Arrhythmia, bradycardia (<50 bpm), or tachycardia [>(230 – age) × 0.8]
  - • Ischemia-induced myocardial failure
  - • Valvular or septal defect
  - • Systemic or pulmonary hypertension
  - • Myocarditis
  - • Myocardiopathies
  - • Elevated right heart/central venous and jugular venous pressure
  - • Decreased cardiac output
  - • Peripheral hypoperfusion
  - • Peripheral edema, pulmonary edema

- ■ Treatment
  - • Opioids relieve pain, provide sedation, block adrenergic discharge
  - • Diuretics decrease vascular volume, decrease right and left atrial pressures
  - • Chronotropic agents are rarely indicated; should be used to raise heart rate only to tolerable levels
  - • Inotropic agents increase blood flow in the cardiovascular system
  - • Vasodilators in patients with elevated systemic vascular resistance
  - • β-Blockers in those with ischemia and a rapid heart rate
  - • Transaortic balloon pump for resuscitating selected patients with severe reversible left ventricular dysfunction

- ■ Pearl

Optimize preload; maximize oxygen; minimize afterload.

Reference

Feliciano DV et al: Advances in the diagnosis and treatment of thoracic trauma. Surg Clin North Am 1999;79:1417.

Hypovolemic Shock

- ■ Essentials of Diagnosis
  - • Inadequate circulating blood volume
  - • Inadequate end-organ perfusion
  - • Hypotension; postural hypotension
  - • Cutaneous vasoconstriction
  - • Sweating
  - • Flat neck veins
  - • Concentrated urine; oliguria
  - • Delayed capillary refill
  - • Thirst
  - • Confusion
  - • Restlessness
  - • Lethargy
  - • Irregular heart rate

- ■ Differential Diagnosis
  - • Hemorrhage
  - • Protracted vomiting
  - • Protracted diarrhea
  - • Fluid sequestration in gut lumen
  - • Loss of plasma into tissues (burns, trauma)

- ■ Treatment
  - • Establish airway
  - • Give nasal oxygen at minimum
  - • Control external hemorrhage
  - • Give 2 L crystalloid wide open for initial resuscitation of severe shock and third liter of crystalloid over 10 minutes
  - • Begin blood transfusion in those who remain unstable after 3 L of crystalloid

- ■ Pearl

Stop bleeding and replace volume before giving pressors.

Reference

Velmahos GC et al: Endpoints of resuscitation of critically injured patients: Normal or supranormal? A prospective randomized trial. Ann Surg 2000;232:409.

Mechanical Pulmonary Failure

- **Essentials of Diagnosis**
  - Hypoxemia
  - Hypercarbia
  - Mechanical insufficiency
  - Chest trauma; chest pain
  - Free-floating chest wall segment
  - Large air leak through wound or chest tube
  - Poor ventilatory effort (pain, debility)
  - Causes include trauma, pain/weakness postoperatively, debility of long-term illness, bronchopleural fistula, hypoxemia

- **Differential Diagnosis**
  - Often has a multifunctional basis, for example a combination of injury, anesthetic, pain medications, and muscle weakness from catabolism
  - All factors must be addressed

- **Treatment**
  - Mechanical ventilation
  - Analgesia
  - Chest tube decompression
  - Chest wall stabilization
  - Occlusion of bronchopleural fistulas
  - Weaning and nutritional support (debility)
  - Tracheostomy (debility)

- **Pearl**

People lose strength fast and gain it only slowly; it is better to keep them from losing it.

References

Esteban A et al: A comparison of four methods of weaning patients from mechanical ventilation. N Engl J Med 1995;332:345.

Tobin MJ: Weaning from mechanical ventilation; what have we learned? Respir Care 2000;45:417.

Pulmonary Edema, Cardiogenic

- **Essentials of Diagnosis**
  - Hypoxemia
  - Rales
  - Post-myocardial infarction
  - Surgical stress or fluid shifts with underlying coronary artery disease
  - Fluid overload
  - Elevated pulmonary artery wedge pressures on pulmonary artery catheterization
  - Chest film shows cephalization of blood flow, Kerley B lines, perihilar infiltrates

- **Differential Diagnosis**
  - Often has a multifunctional basis, for example a combination of injury, anesthetic, hypervolemia, hypoxia, and underlying coronary artery disease
  - All factors must be addressed

- **Treatment**
  - Minimize fluid intake
  - Minimize salt intake
  - Diuresis
  - Supplemental oxygen; intubation and mechanical ventilation
  - Monitor fluid balance
  - Perform serial ABG measurements
  - Monitor for symptomatic improvement
  - Monitor pulmonary capillary wedge pressure
  - Perform serial chest films
  - Prognosis: determined by the cause of cardiac insufficiency

- **Pearl**

Optimize preload; maximize oxygen; minimize afterload.

Reference

Chang MC et al: Redefining cardiovascular performance during resuscitation: Ventricular stroke work, power, and the pressure-volume diagram. J Trauma 1998;45:470.

Pulmonary Edema, Neurogenic

- **Essentials of Diagnosis**
  - Head injury often present, but syndrome usually due to spinal cord damage; rarely occurs with isolated head injury
  - Increased intracranial pressure
  - Caused by pooling of blood in denervated autonomic venules and small veins
  - Hypotension after trauma
  - Warm extremities, sometimes with hyperemia
  - No other evident causes of shock, such as hypovolemic or cardiogenic

- **Differential Diagnosis**
  - Usually due to spinal cord injury; not caused by isolated head injury; perform radiographic evaluation of spinal column
  - Therapeutic test: Trendelenburg position followed by 2 L intravenous (IV) fluid bolus; if shock persists, consider phenylephrine infusion and other causes

- **Treatment**
  - Supportive care of blood pressure to maintain perfusion
  - Stabilize and protect spine from further injury

- **Pearl**

Beware the spinal cord in a warm, hypotensive trauma patient.

Reference

Irish JC et al: Penetrating and blunt neck trauma: 10-year review of a Canadian experience. Can J Surg 1997;40:33.

Septic Shock

- **Essentials of Diagnosis**
  - Infection
  - Either high or low cardiac output
  - Hypotension
  - Low systemic vascular resistance
  - Fever and chills
  - Evidence of infection or perforation
  - Warm, flushed skin
  - Tachycardia
  - Anxiety and confusion

- **Differential Diagnosis**
  - High-output septic shock can be produced by bowel perforation, necrotic intestine, abscesses, gangrene, and soft-tissue infections
  - Cardiovascular findings of low-output sepsis are identical to those of hypovolemic shock
  - Diagnosis is usually clear from clinical circumstances

- **Treatment**
  - Invasive monitoring (pulmonary artery catheter)
  - IV fluid resuscitation
  - Inotropic agents
  - Antibiotics
  - Remove necrotic tissue or debride or drain infection
  - Treatment is determined by the underlying cause

- **Pearl**

Drain the pus.

Reference

Holcroft JW, Wisner DH: Shock & acute pulmonary failure in surgical patients. In Way LW, Doherty GM (editors): Current Surgical Diagnosis & Treatment, 11th ed. McGraw-Hill, 2003.

3

Trauma

Abdominal Injuries

- ■ Essentials of Diagnosis
  - Focused abdominal sonography for trauma (FAST) examination is used to identify abnormal collections of blood or fluid
  - Obviates the need for diagnostic peritoneal lavage

- ■ Differential Diagnosis
  - Computed tomography (CT) has primary role in defining intra-abdominal injuries from blunt trauma; do not obtain CT scan in an unstable patient
  - Diagnostic laparoscopy is useful in penetrating abdominal trauma
  - Exploratory laparotomy has 3 main indications after blunt injury: peritonitis, unexplained hypovolemia, and other injuries known to be associated with intra-abdominal injuries

- ■ Treatment
  - Liver injuries: control hemorrhage at laparotomy; if massive blood loss has occurred before surgery, consider packing the liver and reexploring in 24–48 hours
  - Biliary tract injuries: treat gallbladder injuries with cholecystectomy; 50–80% can be managed nonoperatively
  - Pancreatic injuries: moderate injuries require operative exploration, debridement, and external drains; severe injuries may require distal resection or external drainage
  - Gastrointestinal tract injuries: most treated with lateral repair; some require resection with end-to-end anastomosis
  - Duodenal hematomas: usually resolve nonoperatively; obstruction for >10–14 days may require operative evacuation
  - Colon injuries: divert fecal stream or exteriorize the injury
  - Bladder rupture: frequently associated with pelvic fractures; repair through a midline abdominal incision; divert urine
  - Renal vascular injuries: immediate operation to save the kidney
  - Ureteral injuries: easily missed; reconstruct by primary repair, ureteroureterostomy, or ureteral reimplantation
  - Stab wounds of lower chest or abdomen: most should be explored
  - Gunshot wounds of lower chest and abdomen: all should be explored

- ■ Pearl

Missed injuries kill patients.

Reference

Sartorelli KH et al: Nonoperative management of hepatic, splenic, and renal injuries in adults with multiple injuries. J Trauma 2000;49:56.

Arterial Injuries

- **Essentials of Diagnosis**
  - Penetrating injuries: stab wounds, low-velocity (<2000 ft/s) bullet wounds, iatrogenic injuries, and inadvertent intra-arterial injection of drugs produce less soft-tissue injury and less disruption of collateral circulation; high-velocity missiles produce more extensive vascular injuries, with massive destruction and contamination of surrounding tissues
  - Blunt injuries: especially likely near joints, where vessels are relatively fixed and vulnerable to shear forces
  - Ischemia: must be suspected when patient has one or more of the "5 Ps": pain, pallor, paralysis, paresthesias, pulselessness
  - Arteriovenous fistula: with simultaneous injury of adjacent artery and vein, a fistula may form that allows blood from the artery to enter the vein
  - Workup: physical examination ("5 Ps," bruit, thrill, expanding hematoma), ankle-brachial index bilaterally, arteriography (most accurate), duplex Doppler (noninvasive)

- **Differential Diagnosis**
  - Arterial injury must be considered in any injured patient
  - Diagnosis is usually based on physical examination
  - Look for "5 Ps" and listen for bruit, feel for a thrill, and look for an expanding hematoma

- **Treatment**
  - Initial: repair within 12 hours makes amputation unlikely
  - Operative: at least one uninjured extremity should be prepared for surgery to provide vein if necessary; intraoperative angiography should be available; completion arteriography is always indicated (even with palpable distal pulses)
  - Current recommendations call for repair or shunting of vascular injury before stabilization of associated fracture
  - Fasciotomy is indicated for combined arterial and venous injury, massive soft-tissue damage, delay between injury and repair (4–6 hours), prolonged hypotension, excessive swelling, or high tissue pressure

- **Pearl**

Presence of a pulse distal to the injury does not preclude arterial injury.

References

Asensio JA et al: Operative management and outcome of 302 abdominal vascular injuries. Am J Surg 2000;180:528.

Sparks SR et al: Arterial injury in uncomplicated upper extremity dislocations. Ann Vasc Surg 2000;14:110.

Blast Injury

- **Essentials of Diagnosis**
    - Injuries occur from the effects of the blast itself, propelled foreign bodies, or falling objects
    - Pathophysiology involves 2 mechanisms: crush injury from rapid displacement of the body wall, leading to laceration and contusion of underlying structures; and wave propagation, which transfers energy to internal sites
    - Blast-induced shock may be result of myocardial depression without compensatory circulatory vasoconstriction
    - Perform the ABCs (airway, breathing, circulation) of trauma evaluation; chest film, pelvic x-ray, and abdominal CT scans are useful in stable patients

- **Differential Diagnosis**
    - Must evaluate for associated penetrating trauma

- **Treatment**
    - Severe injuries with shock from blood loss or hypoxia require resuscitative measures
    - Maintain high index of suspicion for hollow organ perforation (especially if victim was submerged at time of blast)

- **Pearl**

Missed injuries kill patients.

Reference

Cernak I et al: Recognizing, scoring and predicting blast injuries. World J Surg 1999;23:44.

Diaphragmatic Hernia, Traumatic

- **Essentials of Diagnosis**
  - May be acute or chronic following either penetrating or blunt trauma
  - Acute form is associated with respiratory distress
  - Chronic form is marked by pain and bowel obstruction
  - Chest film shows a radiopaque area and occasionally an air-fluid level if hollow viscera have herniated
  - If stomach has entered the chest, the abnormal path of a nasogastric tube may be diagnostic
  - Ultrasound, CT scan, and magnetic resonance imaging demonstrate the diaphragmatic rent

- **Differential Diagnosis**
  - In acute trauma, focus attention on life-threatening injury
  - Diaphragmatic hernia may cause respiratory distress
  - In a patient with a history of abdominal trauma and a clinical picture of bowel obstruction, consider missed diaphragmatic hernia

- **Treatment**
  - For acute condition: repair after patient is stabilized or at the same time as other injuries are treated
  - For chronic condition: symptomatic, urgent repair
  - For asymptomatic patients: elective repair

- **Pearl**

Missed injuries kill patients.

Reference

Grover SB, Ratan SK: Simultaneous dual posttraumatic diaphragmatic and abdominal wall hernias. J Trauma 2001;51:583.

Drowning

- ■ Essentials of Diagnosis
    - • Effects of drowning or near drowning are due to hypoxemia and aspiration
    - • Physiologic effects of salt-water aspiration are different from those of fresh-water aspiration: salt-water aspiration produces hypovolemia, hemoconcentration, and hypertonicity but not hemolysis; aspirated fresh water is quickly absorbed across the alveoli and leads to hypervolemia, hypotonicity, hemolysis, and electrolyte abnormalities
    - • Symptoms and signs include hypoxemia, neurologic impairment, or unconsciousness
    - • After restoring ventilation, perform physical examination, chest film, arterial blood gas (ABG) measurements, blood alcohol levels, and drug screen

- ■ Differential Diagnosis
    - • Evaluate for associated injuries (from a dive or fall)
    - • Check for toxic substances (drugs or alcohol)

- ■ Treatment
    - • Restore ventilation immediately
    - • Correct residual hypoxemia, acidosis, and electrolyte abnormalities
    - • Endotracheal intubation and mechanical ventilation are often necessary
    - • Complications: aspiration-related late acute respiratory failure; red cell lysis (hypotonicity) can lead to hemoglobinuria and acute renal failure; neurologic injury related to hypoxia

- ■ Pearl

Missed injuries kill patients.

Reference

De Nicola LK et al: Submersion injuries in children and adults. Crit Care Clin 1997;13:477.

Hepatic Trauma

- ■ Essentials of Diagnosis
  - • Liver is the most commonly injured organ in blunt abdominal trauma and the second most common injury in penetrating abdominal trauma
  - • Symptoms and signs include shock, abdominal pain, distended abdomen, penetrating wounds, ecchymosis
  - • FAST examination shows intraperitoneal fluid, hepatic laceration, or hepatic hematoma
  - • CT shows extravasation of blood, hematoma, laceration, or parenchyma injury; grade is a poor predictor of operative findings
  - • Perform FAST for blunt trauma, CT for blunt trauma, diagnostic peritoneal lavage if patient with blunt trauma is not stable for CT, laparotomy for penetrating trauma

- ■ Differential Diagnosis
  - • Retrohepatic cava or hepatic vein injury
  - • Portal triad injury
  - • Coagulopathy

- ■ Treatment
  - • Indications: shock and positive FAST or diagnostic peritoneal lavage after blunt trauma, penetrating abdominal trauma, possible major vascular injury on CT, continued active bleeding after blunt trauma and absence of coagulopathy
  - • Operation with direct repair of small defects, and packing for hemostasis with return to operating room after 24–48 hours for larger hepatic injuries
  - • Prognosis: 1% mortality for penetrating trauma, 10–20% mortality for blunt trauma, 70% mortality if 3 major organs including liver are involved

- ■ Pearl

Stop bleeding and replace volume before giving pressors.

Reference

Doherty GM, Way LW: Liver & portal venous system. In Way LW, Doherty GM (editors): Current Surgical Diagnosis & Treatment, 11th ed. McGraw-Hill, 2003. (See Table 25-1, Liver Injury Scale.)

Neck Injuries

- ■ Essentials of Diagnosis
    - All neck injuries are potentially life-threatening
    - Penetrating injuries are divided into zones I, II, and III
    - Injuries to the larynx and trachea may be asymptomatic or cause hoarseness, stridor, or dyspnea; severe chest pain and dysphagia with esophageal perforation may appear late

- ■ Differential Diagnosis
    - Zone 1 injuries occur at the thoracic outlet, extending from clavicles to cricoid cartilage; zone I includes proximal carotid arteries, subclavian vessels, major vessels in the chest
    - Zone II injuries occur in the area between the cricoid and the angle of the mandible
    - Zone III injuries occur between the angle of the mandible and the base of the skull

- ■ Treatment
    - Operation is indicated for shock, expanding hematoma, or uncontrolled hemorrhage
    - Arteriography is recommended for patients with zones I and III injuries to help plan operative approach
    - Proximal vascular control in zone I requires thoracotomy
    - Classic approach to zone II injury penetrating the platysma is operative exploration; alternative in zone II can include arteriography or duplex Doppler, rigid endoscopy, and rigid bronchoscopy as well as contrast study of the esophagus to rule out high esophageal injuries that are easily missed on endoscopy, with operation reserved for identified injuries
    - Zone III injuries are difficult to approach and may require disarticulation of the mandible
    - Esophageal injuries should be sutured and drained; systemic antibiotics are indicated
    - Immediate tracheotomy is needed for airway obstruction
    - Tracheal lacerations should be closed after debridement and distal tracheostomy
    - Complications: untreated injury to larynx and trachea can lead to acute airway obstruction, tracheal stenosis, and sepsis; carotid injuries can cause death from hemorrhage, brain damage, and arteriovenous fistula with cardiac decompensation

- ■ Pearl

Never leave a patient with airway injury alone.

Reference

Eddy VA: Zone I Penetrating Neck Injury Study Group: Is routine arteriography mandatory for penetrating injury to zone 1 of the neck? J Trauma 2000;48:208.

Pleural Space Trauma

- **Essentials of Diagnosis**
  - Hemothorax is classified by the amount of blood: minimal, <350 mL; moderate, 350–1500 mL; massive, >1500 mL
  - The rate of bleeding after evacuation of hemothorax is more important than the initial return of blood on placement of the chest tube
  - Pneumothorax occurs with laceration of the lung or chest wall after penetrating or blunt trauma
  - Tension pneumothorax develops when a flap-valve leak allows air to enter the pleural space but not exit
  - Hemothorax: decreased breath sounds, dullness to percussion
  - Pneumothorax: possibly tympany to percussion, decreased breath sounds
  - Tension pneumothorax: tracheal deviation away from affected side, tympany to percussion, decreased breath sounds, hypotension, distended neck veins
  - Perform physical examination, chest film (upright or semi-upright)

- **Differential Diagnosis**
  - Rib fracture
  - Cardiac contusion
  - Pulmonary contusion
  - Associated abdominal injuries

- **Treatment**
  - Hemothorax: in 85% of cases, tube thoracostomy (chest tube) is all the treatment necessary (NOT needle aspiration)
  - Pneumothorax: tube thoracostomy
  - Tension pneumothorax: needle thoracostomy followed by tube thoracostomy

- **Pearl**

Empty the pleura of air and blood early, or pay late.

Reference

Pape HC et al: Appraisal of early evaluation of chest trauma: Development of a standardized scoring system for initial clinical decision-making. J Trauma 2000;49:496.

Pulmonary Contusion

- **Essentials of Diagnosis**
  - Due to sudden parenchymal concussion from blunt trauma or wounding with a high-velocity missile
  - Occurs in 75% of patients with flail chest, but can occur without associated rib fracture
  - Symptoms and signs include thin and blood-tinged secretions, chest pain, restlessness, apprehensiveness, and labored respirations; eventually, dyspnea, cyanosis, tachypnea, and tachycardia develop
  - Chest film shows patchy parenchymal opacification or diffuse linear peribronchial densities; overlying evidence of chest trauma including skeletal injuries

- **Differential Diagnosis**
  - Pneumothorax
  - Hemothorax
  - Cardiac contusion
  - Rib fractures
  - Associated abdominal injuries

- **Treatment**
  - Oxygen; intubation and mechanical ventilation
  - Avoid excessive hydration
  - Chest wall splinting; analgesia
  - Perform serial ABG measurements, serial chest films, physical examination; watch for pneumonia

- **Pearl**

Radiographic findings lag behind clinical findings.

Reference

Cohn SM: Pulmonary contusion: Review of a clinical entity. J Trauma 1997;42:973.

Thoracic Injuries

- **Essentials of Diagnosis**
  - Simple rib fracture is the most common thoracic injury
  - Early deaths are commonly due to airway obstruction, flail chest, open pneumothorax, massive hemothorax, tension pneumothorax, cardiac tamponade
  - Late deaths are due to respiratory failure, sepsis, unrecognized injuries
  - Symptoms and signs include pain on inspiration, decreased ventilation; cyanosis and ashen or gray facies may indicate upper airway obstruction
  - Tracheal shift, dullness to percussion, and absence of breath sounds unilaterally with flat neck veins can indicate massive hemothorax; tracheal shift, tympany to percussion, and absence of breath sounds unilaterally with distended neck veins may indicate tension pneumothorax

- **Differential Diagnosis**
  - Airway obstruction
  - Tension pneumothorax
  - Flail chest
  - Massive hemothorax
  - Cardiac tamponade
  - Open pneumothorax

- **Treatment**
  - Adequate analgesia
  - Intubation and mechanical ventilation as needed
  - Hospital mortality with isolated thoracic injury is 4–8%, but rises to 10–15% with one other organ system involved and to 35% if multiple organs are involved

- **Pearl**

Radiographic findings lag behind clinical findings.

Reference

Feliciano DV et al: Advances in the diagnosis and treatment of thoracic trauma. Surg Clin North Am 1999;79:1417.

Tracheobronchial Injuries

- **Essentials of Diagnosis**
  - Blunt tracheobronchial injuries often result from compression of the airway between the sternum and the vertebral column
  - Penetrating tracheobronchial injuries may occur at any location
  - Symptoms and signs include massive air leak, poor reexpansion after chest tube placement, pneumothorax, pneumomediastinum, pneumothorax that persists after chest tube placement

- **Differential Diagnosis**
  - Rib fracture
  - Pneumothorax
  - Hemothorax
  - Pulmonary contusion
  - Cardiac contusion
  - Cardiac tamponade
  - Associated abdominal injuries

- **Treatment**
  - Resuscitation and stabilization
  - Chest tube
  - Intubation and mechanical ventilation
  - Immediate primary repair for tracheobronchial laceration

- **Pearl**

Never leave a patient with an airway injury alone.

Reference

Feliciano DV et al: Advances in the diagnosis and treatment of thoracic trauma. Surg Clin North Am 1999;79:1417.

Trauma Evaluation

- **Essentials of Diagnosis**
  - Identify and treat immediate life-threatening conditions; primary evaluation includes airway, breathing, circulation, disability, environment; additional injuries
  - Blood should be drawn immediately for hematocrit, white blood cell count, creatinine, blood urea nitrogen, and blood typing and cross-match
  - ABG measurement should be done if any sign of respiratory compromise
  - Films of the chest and abdomen are required in all major injuries; cervical spine films should be obtained in patients at risk
  - Airway: establishing an adequate airway has the highest priority in the primary survey
  - Breathing: ensure that ventilation is adequate
  - Circulation: gross hemorrhage from accessible wounds is usually obvious and controlled with direct pressure and elevation

- **Differential Diagnosis**
  - Multiple injuries may be identified
  - Address injuries with the ABC approach

- **Treatment**
  - Hypovolemic shock: keep patient recumbent; give balanced salt solution rapidly until signs of shock abate and urinary output normalizes
  - Neurogenic shock: due to pooling of blood in autonomically denervated venules and usually due to spinal cord injury, NOT isolated head injury
  - Treatment priorities: if signs of hypovolemic shock, coma is likely due to cerebral ischemia; resuscitate and replace blood volume first
  - Deepening stupor in patients under observation should arouse suspicion of expanding intracranial lesion
  - Emergency thoracotomy is indicated for cardiopulmonary arrest as a result of penetrating trauma

- **Pearl**

Remember ABCDE: airway, breathing, circulation, disability, environment.

Reference

ATLS Student Manual, 7th ed. American College of Surgeons, 2003.

Burns & Thermal Injury

Burns

- ■ **Essentials of Diagnosis**
  - First-degree burn: involves only epidermis; characterized by erythema and minor microscopic changes; tissue damage is minimal; pain, the chief symptom, usually resolves in 48–72 hours and healing takes place uneventfully
  - Second-degree (partial-thickness) burn: deeper, involving all of the epidermis and some dermis; systemic severity and quality of healing are related to amount of undamaged dermis
  - Complications are rare from superficial partial-thickness burns, which usually heal in 10–14 days
  - Deep partial-thickness burns heal over 25–35 days with a fragile epithelial covering that arises from uninjured epithelium of the deep dermal sweat glands and hair follicles; severe hypertrophic scarring occurs during healing; evaporative losses remain high; conversion to full thickness by bacteria is common

- ■ **Differential Diagnosis**
  - Always evaluate for associated blunt or inhalation injuries

- ■ **Treatment**
  - Administer oxygen
  - If burns are >20% of total body surface area (TBSA), place a Foley catheter to monitor urine output
  - Obtain large-bore intravenous (IV) access, preferably in peripheral vein; central access is associated with infection in burn patients
  - Rough estimate of fluid requirement is 4 mL/% TBSA/kg with 50% given over first 8 hours and remainder over next 16 hours
  - Give tetanus toxoid, 0.5 mL, to all patients with significant burn injury
  - Pain, hypothermia, and anxiety all need aggressive control
  - Begin nutritional support as early as possible to maximize wound healing and minimize immune deficiency
  - Rapid closure of burn wounds decreases sepsis and, in full-thickness burns >60% of TBSA, significantly decreases the death rate
  - Silver sulfadiazine is effective against a wide spectrum of gram-negative organisms and may penetrate burn eschar

- ■ **Pearl**

Early excision and wound coverage speed recovery.

Reference

Nguyen T et al: Current treatment of severely burned patients. Ann Surg 1996;223:14.

Burns, Respiratory Injury

- **Essentials of Diagnosis**
  - Major cause of death after burns is respiratory tract injury
  - Problems include inhalation injury, aspiration, bacterial pneumonia, pulmonary edema, pulmonary embolism, post-traumatic pulmonary insufficiency
  - Direct inhalation injuries are divided into 3 categories: heat injury to the airway, carbon monoxide poisoning, and inhalation of noxious gases
  - Heat injury is rare below the vocal cords
  - Carbon monoxide poisoning must be considered in every patient; arterial blood gas and carboxyhemoglobin (COHb) levels must be measured; COHb >5% in nonsmokers and >10% in smokers indicates carbon monoxide poisoning
  - Severe carbon monoxide poisoning (40–60% COHb) produces hallucinations, confusion, ataxia, collapse, and coma; levels >60% COHb are usually fatal
  - Inhalation of toxic chemicals produces specific respiratory injuries, with severe mucosal edema followed by sloughing
  - Direct laryngoscopy is probably as helpful as fiberoptic laryngoscopy

- **Differential Diagnosis**
  - Inhalation injury, aspiration
  - Bacterial pneumonia
  - Pulmonary edema, pulmonary embolism
  - Post-traumatic pulmonary insufficiency

- **Treatment**
  - All patients require humidified oxygen in high concentration; if carbon monoxide poisoning has occurred, give 100% oxygen until COHb returns to normal and symptoms resolve
  - Corticosteroids are contraindicated
  - Treatment of heat injury below the vocal cords is primarily supportive with pulmonary toilet, mechanical ventilation (as needed), and antibiotics

- **Pearl**

Intubate and bronchoscope early to avoid problems later.

Reference

Nguyen T et al: Current treatment of severely burned patients. Am Surg 1996;223:14.

Electrical Injury

- **Essentials of Diagnosis**
  - Three kinds of electrical injuries occur: current injury, electrothermal burns from arcing current, and flame burns from ignited clothing
  - Damage from electrical current is directly proportional to its intensity (Ohm's law): Amperage = voltage/resistance
  - Current path through the body depends on resistance: bone > fat > tendon > skin > muscle > blood > nerve
  - Skin burn is usually depressed gray or yellow area of full-thickness burn with surrounding hyperemia; charring may be present if arc injury coexists
  - Always transfer patients with significant electrical injuries to specialized centers after initial resuscitation

- **Differential Diagnosis**
  - Always evaluate for associated blunt injury

- **Treatment**
  - All dead and devitalized tissue must be debrided
  - Second debridement is often indicated 24–48 hours after the injury

- **Pearl**

Skin injury shows only the entry and exit points; burn injuries can extend along the internal current path.

Reference

Haberal M: An eleven year survey of electrical burn injuries. J Burn Care Rehabil 1995;16:43.

Frostbite

- **Essentials of Diagnosis**
  - Caused by cold exposure, but effects can be amplified by moisture or wind
  - Ice crystals form between cells and grow at the expense of extracellular fluid; tissue injury is caused by cellular dehydration and ischemia due to vasoconstriction and increased viscosity
  - Frostbitten parts are numb, painless, and white or waxy in appearance; superficial frostbite is compressible with pressure (unfrozen deep tissues); deep frostbite is woody (frozen deep tissues)

- **Differential Diagnosis**
  - After rewarming, frostbitten area becomes mottled blue or purple, painful, and tender
  - Blisters appear that may take weeks to heal

- **Treatment**
  - Frostbitten part should be rewarmed in a water bath at 40–42.2°C for 20–30 minutes; thawing should not be attempted until the victim can be kept permanently warm and at rest
  - Skin should be gently debrided by immersion in a whirlpool for 20 minutes twice daily
  - Vasodilating agents and sympathectomy are NOT helpful; expectant management is the rule
  - Tissue usually sloughs spontaneously; amputation is rarely indicated before 2 months
  - Prognosis: excellent if appropriate treatment is provided; recovered patients have increased susceptibility to future frostbite

- **Pearl**

Debride and amputate late to preserve maximum tissue.

Reference

Peng RY, Bongard FS: Hypothermia in trauma patients. J Am Coll Surg 1999;188:685.

Heatstroke

- ■ Essentials of Diagnosis
  - Occurs when body core temperature exceeds 40°C and produces severe central nervous system dysfunction
  - Result of imbalance between heat production and dissipation
  - Kills approximately 4000 persons each year in the United States
  - Predisposing factors include dermatitis, use of phenothiazines, β-blockers, diuretics, and anticholinergics; unrelated fever; obesity; alcoholism; heavy clothing
  - Symptoms and signs include sudden coma in hot environment; prodrome of dizziness, headache, nausea, chills, and gooseflesh of arms and chest rarely seen; heart rate of 140–170 bpm; hyperventilation may reach 60 breaths per minute with respiratory alkalosis; pulmonary edema and bloody sputum in severe cases

- ■ Differential Diagnosis
  - Dehydration
  - Cerebrovascular accident
  - Myocardial infarction
  - Drug overdose; alcohol intoxication or poisoning

- ■ Treatment
  - Patient should be cooled rapidly: spraying patient with water that is 15°C and fanning with warm air are most efficient; immersion in ice-water bath is often needed
  - Administer oxygen
  - Intubate as needed for PaO_2 <65 mm Hg
  - Give IV mannitol early if myoglobinuria is present
  - Patients with disseminated intravascular coagulation may require hemodialysis
  - Bad prognostic indicators include temperature >42.2°C, coma >2 hours, shock, hyperkalemia, aspartate aminotransferase >1000 U/L in first 24 hours
  - Mortality is 10% in those treated promptly

- ■ Pearl

Cool rapidly, rehydrate, and protect the kidneys.

Reference

Bouchama A, DeVol EB: Acid-base alterations in heatstroke. Intensive Care Med 2001;27:680.

Hypothermia, Accidental

■ Essentials of Diagnosis

- Uncontrolled lowering of core body temperature to <35°C by exposure to cold
- Ethyl alcohol facilitates hypothermia by producing sedation (which inhibits shivering) and cutaneous dilation
- Patient appears mentally depressed (somnolent, stuporous, or comatose), cold, pale, or cyanotic; has slow and shallow respirations; is usually normotensive and bradycardic
- At temperatures <32°C, shivering is absent and patient may appear dead

■ Differential Diagnosis

- Patients should never be considered dead until all measures for resuscitation have failed and the patient has been rewarmed

■ Treatment

- Active rewarming is indicated for temperatures <32°C, cardiovascular instability, or failure of passive rewarming
- Methods for rewarming include immersion in warm water, inhalation of heated air, pleural and peritoneal lavage, extracorporeal blood warming
- Partial cardiopulmonary bypass is the most efficient technique and is indicated for ventricular fibrillation, severe hypothermia, or frozen extremities
- Monitor body temperature continuously
- Prognosis: 50% of patients survive when core temperature is <32.2°C; coexisting disease (stroke, myocardial infarction, cancer) increases mortality to 75% or more
- Death may result from pneumonitis, heart failure, or acute renal failure

■ Pearl

Only dead once warm and dead.

Reference

Peng RY, Bongard FS: Hypothermia in trauma patients. J Am Coll Surg 1999;188:685.

Surgical Infections

Actinomycosis & Nocardiosis

■ **Essentials of Diagnosis**

- Actinomycosis: *Actinomyces israelii* is a gram-positive, non-acid-fast, filamentous anaerobic organism that usually shows branching and may break up into short bacterial forms, part of the normal flora of the human oropharynx and upper intestinal tract
- Chronic, slowly progressive infection may involve many tissues, resulting in granulomas and abscesses that drain through sinuses and fistulas; pus contains "sulfur granules"; lesions are often hard, relatively painless, and nontender
- Nocardiosis: nocardiae are gram-positive, aerobic, branching, filamentous, and may be acid-fast; *Nocardia asteroides* is the most common isolate
- May present in two forms: (1) localized, chronic granuloma with suppuration, abscess, and sinus tract formation resembling actinomycosis; (2) systemic infection, usually beginning as pneumonitis with suppuration and progressing via the bloodstream to involve other organs
- Systemic infection produces fever, cough, and weight loss and resembles mycobacterial or mycotic infections
- Actinomycosis and nocardiosis are not communicable

■ **Differential Diagnosis**

- Chronic wounds that do not heal because of mechanical issues such as scars

■ **Treatment**

- Actinomycosis is treated with penicillin G for many weeks
- Nocardiosis is best treated with sulfonamides or, when severe, with imipenem plus amikacin for many weeks
- Surgery may be indicated to drain abscesses, excise fistulas, repair defects or involved organs
- Prognosis: mortality rate of nocardial bacteremia reaches 50%

■ **Pearl**

Consider actinomycosis for chronic draining sinuses.

References

Lerner PI: Nocardiosis. Clin Infect Dis 1996;22:891.
Smego R Jr et al: Actinomycosis. Clin Infect Dis 1998;26:1255.

Bites, Arthropod

- ■ Essentials of Diagnosis
  - Some arthropod bites are fatal because of direct toxicity or hypersensitivity reactions
  - Bite of the Latrodectus species of black widow (*Latrodectus mactans*) or the red-backed spider (*Latrodectus hasseltii*) has primarily systemic neurotoxic effects; the brown recluse spider (*Loxosceles recluse*) is dark tan and has a violin-shaped mark on the back of the main body; bites cause tissue necrosis
  - Latrodectism: symptoms of envenomation begin with pain at the bite location followed by abdominal pain and cramping, respiratory difficulty, and potential paralysis
  - Loxoscelism: bite may cause local signs of erythema and edema but usually minimal pain; hemorrhagic bullae surrounded by localized ischemia develop over the next 24–48 hours

- ■ Differential Diagnosis
  - Tetanus
  - Clostridial infections
  - Bacterial infection of puncture wound

- ■ Treatment
  - After a bee sting, apply ice packs early to reduce swelling; elevate the extremity
  - Loxoscelism is managed by supportive measures; infected bites may require operative debridement
  - Bee and wasp stings: if a severe or anaphylactic reaction occurs, aqueous epinephrine (0.5–1 mL of 1:1000 solution) should be given intramuscularly; oxygen, plasma expanders, and pressor agents may be required in case of shock; intravenous (IV) calcium gluconate may relieve pain and spasm
  - Loxoscelism: corticosteroids or dapsone (50–100 mg/d) may be indicated if ulcers develop or the local reaction progresses rapidly

- ■ Pearl

Bees and wasps kill more people than any other venomous animal.

Reference

Bond GR: Snake, spider, and scorpion envenomation in North America. Pediatr Rev 1999;20:147.

Cellulitis

■ Essentials of Diagnosis

- Common invasive, nonsuppurative infection of connective tissue
- Diffuse inflammation without signs of necrotizing infection
- Most often caused by group A streptococci and *Staphylococcus aureus*
- Symptoms and signs include brawny red or reddish-brown area of edematous skin; moderate or high fever is almost always present; warm, erythematous, edematous area; lymphangitis produces red, warm, tender streaks 3–4 mm wide leading from the infection along lymphatic vessels
- Blood cultures are positive in only 2% of cases; needle aspiration yields positive cultures only 20–40% of the time

■ Differential Diagnosis

- Hemorrhagic bullae and skin necrosis suggest necrotizing fasciitis
- Complete history and physical examination should help to distinguish inciting factors
- History of open wound, break in the skin, or puncture

■ Treatment

- Rest, elevation, warm packs, and an oral or IV antibiotic; penicillins or first-generation cephalosporins are given IV
- If a clear response has not occurred in 12–24 hours, suspect abscess or consider whether the causative agent is a gram-negative rod or resistant organism

■ Pearl

Lack of improvement implies underlying abscess.

Reference

Cobb JP et al: Inflammation, infection, & antibiotics. In Way LW, Doherty GM (editors): Current Surgical Diagnosis & Treatment, 11th ed. McGraw-Hill, 2003.

Echinococcosis

- **Essentials of Diagnosis**
  - Hydatid disease caused by the microscopic cestode parasites *Echinococcus granulosus* and *Echinococcus multilocularis*
  - Foxes, coyotes, dogs, and cats are the definitive hosts that harbor the adult tapeworms in their intestines
  - Ova penetrate the intestine and pass via the portal vein to the liver (75%) and then to the lung (15%) or other tissues; ovum typically develops into a cyst filled with clear fluid; 80% of hydatid cysts are single and in the right lobe
  - Eosinophilia is present in about 40% of patients
  - Perform Casoni skin test; ultrasound and computed tomography reveal calcification and daughter cysts within the parent cyst

- **Differential Diagnosis**
  - Benign hepatic cysts
  - Bacterial or amebic liver abscess
  - Hepatic tumor

- **Treatment**
  - Surgery: remove any cysts without disseminating the organism; excise the intact cyst
  - Medications: albendazole, praziquantel, mebendazole; scolicidal agent (hypertonic sodium chloride solution or sodium hypochlorite solution) can be placed in the cyst
  - Complications: cholangitis, biliary obstruction, rupture into the peritoneal cavity, anaphylaxis

- **Pearl**

Protect against spilling the cyst contents.

Reference

Taylor BR et al: Current surgical management of hepatic cyst disease. Adv Surg 1997;31:127.

Furuncle, Carbuncle, & Hidradenitis Suppurativa

- **Essentials of Diagnosis**
  - Furuncles and carbuncles: cutaneous abscesses that begin in skin glands and hair follicles
  - Furuncles (boils) usually start in infected hair follicles; some are caused by retained foreign bodies and injuries
  - Furuncles itch and cause pain; skin first becomes red and then turns white and necrotic over the top of the abscess
  - Carbuncle is a deep-seated mass of fistulous tracts between infected hair follicles
  - Carbuncles start as furuncles, with infection dissecting through the dermis and subcutaneous tissue in connecting tunnels; extensions open to the surface, giving the appearance of large furuncles with many pustular openings
  - Staphylococci and anaerobic diphtheroids are the most common organisms
  - Hidradenitis suppurativa is a serious skin infection of the axillae or groin consisting of multiple abscesses of the apocrine sweat glands

- **Differential Diagnosis**
  - Actinomycosis
  - Squamous cell skin cancer
  - Sebaceous cyst
  - Rheumatoid nodules
  - Gout
  - Bursitis
  - Erythema nodosum

- **Treatment**
  - Drain abscesses; treat invasive carbuncles by excision and antibiotics; extensively launder all clothing
  - Hidradenitis is usually treated by drainage of the individual abscess followed by careful hygiene; apocrine sweat-bearing skin must be excised; if the deficit is large, closure with a skin graft may be indicated; use of antibiotics depends on location of the abscess and extent of infection; without adequate excision, hidradenitis may become chronic and disabling

- **Pearl**

Personal hygiene is a good thing.

Reference

Brown TJ et al: Hidradenitis suppurativa. South Med J 1998;91:1107.

Herpes Zoster

- **Essentials of Diagnosis**
  - Herpes zoster is an acute vesicular eruption due to reactivation of the varicella-zoster virus
  - Symptoms and signs include focal, often severe, unilateral abdominal wall pain that upon careful questioning follows a dermatomal distribution; delayed development (>48 hours) of classic vesicular lesions along a specific dermatomal distribution
  - Usually occurs in adults
  - With rare exceptions, patients suffer only one attack
  - Obtain dermatology consult to diagnose herpetic rash and perform Tzanck smear

- **Differential Diagnosis**
  - Nerve compression
  - Cellulitis
  - Wound infection

- **Treatment**
  - Exclude surgical cause of abdominal wall pain
  - Evaluate for human immunodeficiency virus or other immunocompromised states in patients <55 years
  - Medications: acyclovir, famciclovir, or valacyclovir; early medical treatment of zoster may reduce the incidence of postherpetic neuralgia (controversial)
  - Prognosis: postherpetic neuralgia develops in 15% of patients

- **Pearl**

Severe pain preceding rash implies zoster.

Reference

Balfour HH: Antiviral drugs. N Engl J Med 1999;340:1255.

Necrotizing Fasciitis

- **Essentials of Diagnosis**
  - Usually caused by multiple bacterial pathogens, including streptococci, staphylococci, anaerobes, gram-negative aerobes
  - Typically begins in localized area (puncture wound, incision) and spreads along fascial planes; results in thrombosis of penetrating vessels and tissue necrosis; area of fascial necrosis usually more extensive than skin appearance indicates
  - Symptoms and signs include hemorrhagic bullae; crepitus may be present; skin may be anesthetic, edematous; patient may have fever, pain, tachycardia; undermining and dissection of the subcutaneous tissue, liquefaction of fat, preservation of overlying skin; "dishwater" exudate from wound; skin necrosis and gangrene in advanced disease; elevated white blood cell count; positive wound culture and Gram stain
  - Biopsy of infected tissue reveals necrosis, polymorphonuclear leukocyte infiltration, thrombi of arteries and veins passing through fascia, angiitis

- **Differential Diagnosis**
  - Cellulitis
  - Soft tissue abscess

- **Treatment**
  - Wide surgical debridement is mainstay of therapy
  - IV broad-spectrum antibiotics: penicillin + aminoglycoside + clindamycin or imipenem-cilastatin; may need to change antibiotics based on wound cultures and sensitivities
  - Wounds may require further debridement either at bedside or in operating room
  - Prognosis: 20% mortality with necrotizing fasciitis; >50% mortality with streptococcal toxic shock syndrome; mortality doubles when >24 hours elapse between diagnosis and operation

- **Pearl**

Skin bullae in a diabetic patient are a surgical emergency.

Reference

Cobb JP et al: Inflammation, infection, & antibiotics. In Way LW, Doherty GM (editors): Current Surgical Diagnosis & Treatment, 11th ed. McGraw-Hill, 2003.

Pilonidal Disease

- **Essentials of Diagnosis**
    - Acute, chronic, recurring abscess or chronic draining sinus over the sacrococcygeal or perianal region
    - Acquired infection of natal cleft hair follicles that become distended and obstructed and rupture into the subcutaneous tissues to form a pilonidal abscess; hair from the surrounding skin is pulled into the abscess cavity by friction generated by the gluteal muscles during walking
    - Most common in hirsute, moderately obese patients
    - Symptoms and signs include pain, fluctuant mass, tenderness, purulent drainage

- **Differential Diagnosis**
    - Perianal abscess
    - Fistula in ano
    - Necrotizing fasciitis

- **Treatment**
    - Drain abscess under local anesthesia; insert probe into the primary opening and unroof the abscess; pull out granulation tissue and inspissated hair; excise with open packing, marsupialization, or primary closure with or without flaps
    - Prevention: meticulous skin care (shaving of natal cleft), perineal hygiene, wound cleansing

- **Pearl**

Minimize the cleft and hair to prevent recurrence.

Reference

Spivak H et al: Treatment of chronic pilonidal disease. Dis Colon Rectum 1996;39:1136.

Rabies

- ■ Essentials of Diagnosis
  - Viral (ssRNA rhabdovirus) encephalitis of mammals transmitted through the saliva of an infected animal; humans are usually inoculated by the bite of a rabid bat, raccoon, skunk, fox, or other wild animal
  - 30% of victims have no memory or evidence of a bite
  - Clinical symptoms begin with pain and numbness around the site of the wound; nonspecific flulike symptoms of fever, irritability, malaise; and progressive cerebral dysfunction
  - Direct fluorescent antibody test on brain tissue is used most frequently to diagnose rabies in animals; serum and cerebrospinal fluid are tested for antibodies; any animal suspected of being rabid should be killed and its brain studied

- ■ Differential Diagnosis
  - Rabies virus has distinctive bullet shape and nonsegmented, negative-stranded RNA genome
  - Rule out cellulitis, abscess, bacterial wound infection, flu

- ■ Treatment
  - Because established disease is almost invariably fatal, early prevention is essential
  - Prevention: wound should be washed thoroughly with soap and water; rabies prophylaxis has proved nearly 100% successful
  - Medications: human rabies immune globulin, human diploid cell vaccine

- ■ Pearl

Get the animal or take the prophylaxis.

Reference

Centers for Disease Control and Prevention, National Center for Infectious Diseases: http://www.cdc.gov/ncidod/dvrd/rabies

Snakebite

- **Essentials of Diagnosis**
  - Distinguishing whether the patient has been bitten and envenomed, bitten but not envenomed, or bitten by a nonvenomous snake is critical before starting treatments
  - A bite by a venomous snake results in envenomation in only 50–70% of cases; indigenous venomous snakes of North America include rattlesnake, copperhead, cottonmouth, and coral snake; pit vipers include rattlesnakes, copperhead, and cottonmouth
  - Hemotoxic effects are mediated by proteolytic enzymes, peptides, and metalloproteins that cause local tissue destruction directly and by intimal injury to blood vessels, followed by thrombosis and necrosis; activation of the coagulation cascade can occur at multiple points, resulting in net anticoagulation
  - Bites by coral snakes lack the characteristic fang marks of bites by pit vipers
  - Symptoms and signs include severe pain, hypotension, diaphoresis, nausea, weakness, and faintness; perioral or peripheral paresthesias, taste changes, and fasciculations
  - Neurotoxic venom can cause dysphagia, dysphonia, diplopia, headache, weakness, and respiratory distress
  - Most snake bites in the United States are from nonvenomous snakes; identification of the snake is helpful

- **Differential Diagnosis**
  - Venomous or non-venomous snake bite; scorpion sting, bee, wasp, or hornet sting; spider bite; puncture wound

- **Treatment**
  - Tourniquets, wound incision and suction, application of ice, cryotherapy, electrical shock, and ingestion of alcohol have no proven value
  - Local wound management includes cleansing and disinfection
  - Specific antivenins are available for the bites of pit vipers and Eastern coral snakes; crotalidae polyvalent antivenin is most effective when given within 4 hours after a bite, of less value after 8 hours, and of questionable value after 30 hours
  - Administer antivenin early as a dilute continuous IV infusion
  - Complications: acute hemolytic anemia, acute tubular necrosis

- **Pearl**

Coral snakes: red on black, venom lack; red on yellow, kill a fellow.

Reference

Chippaux JP et al: Venoms, antivenoms and immunotherapy. Toxicon 1998;36:823.

Surgical Site Infections

- ■ Essentials of Diagnosis
  - Postoperative wound infections resulting from bacterial contamination during or after a surgical procedure
  - Infection usually is confined to the subcutaneous tissues
  - Infection is more likely if: excessive tissue trauma, undrained hematoma, retained foreign bodies, excessively tight ligatures, wound desiccation, poor perfusion, poor oxygenation, dead space
  - Degree of intraoperative contamination is divided into 4 categories that correlate with risk of postoperative wound infection: (1) clean: no gross contamination from exogenous or endogenous sources; (2) clean-contaminated: for example, with gastric or biliary surgery; (3) heavily contaminated: operations on the unprepared colon or emergency operations for intestinal bleeding or perforation; and (4) infected
  - Infection frequency: clean, 1.5%; clean-contaminated, 2–5%; heavily contaminated, 5–30%; infected, 100%
  - Classification of surgical site infections: incisional, superficial (skin and subcutaneous tissues), and deep incisional (deep soft tissue of the incision); organ/space infection: any part of the anatomy other than body wall
  - Infection usually appears between the fifth and tenth postoperative days, but may appear as early as day 1

- ■ Differential Diagnosis
  - Cellulitis
  - Herpes zoster
  - Subcutaneous fat necrosis

- ■ Treatment
  - Mild superficial wound infections: IV antibiotics
  - Deep wound infections: drainage; remove a few staples or stitches and break up the abscess with a sterile cotton-tip swab
  - Antibiotic prophylaxis: choose antibiotics effective against the expected type of contamination; use only if the risk of infection justifies doing so; give at appropriate doses and times; stop dosing before side effects outweigh benefits

- ■ Pearl

Undrained pus won't respond to antibiotics.

References

Centers for Disease Control and Prevention, Division of Healthcare Quality Promotion: http://www.cdc.gov/ncidod/hip

Culver DH et al: Surgical wound infection rates by wound class, operative procedure, and patient risk index. National Nosocomial Infections Surveillance System. Am J Med 1991;91:152S.

Tetanus

- **Essentials of Diagnosis**
  - Anaerobic infection complicated by a neurotoxin that causes nervous irritability and tetanic muscular contraction
  - Causative organism is *Clostridium tetani* in wounds contaminated with soil or feces
  - Occurrence of tetanus in United States has dropped over the last 5 decades; disproportionate number of cases (35%) is reported in persons aged ≥60 years who are unvaccinated or inadequately vaccinated
  - Symptoms of tetanus may occur as soon as 1 day after exposure or as long as several months later; spasms of the facial muscles (risus sardonicus), neck stiffness, dysphagia
  - Wound isolation of the organism is neither sensitive nor specific; perform history and physical examination; careful examination of wound; determine tetanus prophylaxis status

- **Differential Diagnosis**
  - Bacterial wound infection
  - Envenomation

- **Treatment**
  - All patients with traumatic wounds must be asked about tetanus prophylaxis
  - Neutralization of the toxin with tetanus immune globulin
  - IV high-dose penicillin
  - Ventilator support if indicated
  - Surgical wound debridement
  - Each person should be immunized with tetanus toxoid, beginning with routine childhood immunization and continuing with booster injections every 10 years

- **Pearl**

Assess tetanus immunization status in all patients with penetrating wounds.

Reference

Centers for Disease Control and Prevention: Practice Guidelines. http://www.cdc.gov/nip/publications/pin

Section II

Acute Abdomen & Hernias

Chapters

Acute Abdomen

Appendiceal Neoplasms

- ■ Essentials of Diagnosis
  - Most diagnosed during appendectomy for acute appendicitis; some discovered incidentally during other abdominal procedures
  - Mucin secretion from peritoneal cystadenocarcinoma implants is a cause of pseudomyxoma peritonei
  - Incidence: 4.6% of benign tumors in appendectomy specimens; 1.4% of malignant tumors in appendectomy specimens
  - Malignant tumors include carcinoid, mucinous cystadenocarcinoma, and adenocarcinoma; diagnosis is virtually never made preoperatively
  - Clinical presentation in small portion of patients is carcinoid syndrome or widespread metastases; patients with carcinoid syndrome may have elevations of 5-hydroxyindoleacetic acid
  - Radiographic findings are usually consistent with acute appendicitis (enlarged appendix with periappendiceal fat stranding on computed tomography [CT]); most diagnoses depend on pathologic evaluation of the appendiceal specimen; abdominal or pelvic CT scan is used to evaluate for metastatic disease; somatostatin receptor scintigraphy can be helpful with carcinoid tumors; up to 35% of patients with adenocarcinoma have a second gastrointestinal (GI) malignancy

- ■ Differential Diagnosis
  - Acute appendicitis, appendiceal abscess, carcinoid mucinous cystadenoma
  - Rule out synchronous carcinoid neoplasms, metastatic disease

- ■ Treatment
  - Carcinoids <2 cm: appendectomy alone
  - Carcinoids >2 cm or with mucinous elements or invasion of the mesoappendix or cecum: right hemicolectomy
  - All (nonmetastatic) adenocarcinoma: right hemicolectomy
  - Prognosis: very good for benign lesions and small carcinoids; adenocarcinoma has 5-year survival of 60% after right hemicolectomy

- ■ Pearl

Always check the pathology report after appendectomy.

Reference

Way L: Appendix. In Way LW, Doherty GM (editors): Current Surgical Diagnosis & Treatment, 11th ed. McGraw-Hill, 2003.

Appendicitis, Acute

- **Essentials of Diagnosis**
  - About 7% of people in Western countries have appendicitis at some time in their lives; 200,000 appendectomies for acute appendicitis are performed each year in the United States
  - Pathophysiology: occlusion of the proximal lumen by fibrous bands, lymphoid hyperplasia, fecaliths, calculi, or parasites
  - Symptoms classically include abdominal pain before nausea and vomiting; pain is periumbilical initially, then localizes to right lower quadrant
  - Signs include right lower quadrant rebound or percussion tenderness (localized "peritoneal irritation"), mild leukocytosis (10–15 K/mm^3) with left shift
  - Spiral CT (abdominal/pelvic or dedicated "appendiceal protocol") is most sensitive and specific radiographic test; obtain CT scans for atypical clinical presentation or laboratory findings

- **Differential Diagnosis**
  - Genitourinary: acute salpingitis, pelvic inflammatory disease (PID), dysmenorrhea, ovarian lesions, urinary tract infections (UTIs)
  - GI: regional enteritis or complicated Crohn disease, viral gastroenterologic infection, mesenteric adenitis, mesenteric ischemia, small bowel obstruction, cecal volvulus, right-sided diverticulitis
  - Other: incarcerated hernia, acute cholecystitis, complicated peptic ulcer disease

- **Treatment**
  - CT scan or 24-hour admission for serial abdominal examinations or diagnostic laparoscopy for "nonclassic" presentation
  - Appendectomy can be performed open or laparoscopically; interval appendectomy for patients with right lower quadrant abscess who were treated initially with percutaneous drainage
  - Prophylactic antibiotics are indicated preoperatively only for nonperforated disease
  - Complications include wound infection or right lower quadrant abscess (up to 30% in perforated appendicitis)

- **Pearl**

Uncommon presentations of appendicitis are more frequent than most other causes of abdominal symptoms.

Reference

Anderson RE et al: Repeated clinical and laboratory examinations in patients with an equivocal diagnosis of appendicitis. World J Surg 2000;24:479.

Ectopic Pregnancy, Ruptured

- ■ Essentials of Diagnosis
  - • Symptoms and signs include severe abdominal tenderness with guarding, hemodynamic instability, adnexal mass
  - • At least 2 in every 100 pregnancies are ectopic; 95% of ectopic pregnancies occur in the uterine tube, usually the ampullary portion
  - • Risk factors include prior ectopic pregnancy, history of PID, prior pelvic surgery, current intrauterine device use, smoking, diethylstilbestrol exposure, increasing age; in vitro fertilization has increased the incidence of heterotopic pregnancy (intrauterine + ectopic)
  - • Findings include positive β-human chorionic gonadotropin (β-hCG); transvaginal ultrasound is the radiographic procedure of choice

- ■ Differential Diagnosis
  - • Threatened abortion
  - • Missed abortion
  - • Other causes of abdominal pain

- ■ Treatment
  - • Treatment is operative; all patients with ruptured ectopic pregnancy require immediate laparotomy
  - • Complications: infertility, repeat ectopic pregnancy
  - • Prognosis: mortality is 0.3% in ectopic pregnancy

- ■ Pearl

Perform a pregnancy test in every woman of childbearing age with abdominal symptoms.

Reference

Lehner R et al: Ectopic pregnancy. Arch Gynecol Obstet 2000;263:87.

Intra-abdominal Abscess

- ■ Essentials of Diagnosis
  - • Symptoms and signs include fever and chills, tachycardia, leukocytosis, bacteremia, focal abdominal tenderness
  - • Most common causes are GI perforation, postoperative complications, penetrating trauma, genitourinary infections
  - • Broadly classified based on anatomic location: subdiaphragmatic, subhepatic, pericolic, pelvic, interloop
  - • Abdominal pelvic CT scan with intravenous (IV) and oral contrast is the best diagnostic study with >95% sensitivity, particularly in postoperative patients; percutaneous drainage can often be performed at the same setting
  - • Also perform complete blood count (CBC), blood cultures

- ■ Differential Diagnosis
  - • Other causes of abdominal pain and fever: appendicitis, diverticulitis, cholecystitis, mesenteric vascular occlusion, UTI

- ■ Treatment
  - • IV antibiotic therapy initially for small abscesses of <1–2 cm if patient is clinically stable
  - • For most abscesses, prompt and complete drainage, control of the primary cause, and adjunctive use of antibiotics; success rate is 80% for simple abscesses but <50% for complex multiloculated abscesses
  - • Operative indications: percutaneously inaccessible abscesses, persistent focus of infection such as anastomotic leak or perforated diverticulitis, failure of percutaneous drainage
  - • Initially, empiric IV antibiotic coverage for enteric aerobic and anaerobic organisms; subsequently, focused antibiotic therapy based on culture results
  - • Satisfactory drainage achieves clinical improvement within 48–72 hours; serial ultrasound or CT evaluations sometimes obtained to verify cavity obliteration
  - • Prognosis: mortality for serious intra-abdominal abscesses is about 30%

- ■ Pearl

Drain the pus to improve the patient's condition.

Reference

Farthmann EH, Schoffel U: Epidemiology and pathophysiology of intraabdominal infections (IAI). Infection 1998;26:329.

Pain, Abdominal, Nonspecific

■ Essentials of Diagnosis

- Diagnosis of exclusion: abdominal pain with no identifiable organic pathology
- Common features include improvement or no change in abdominal pain since onset of symptoms and lack of associated serious signs or symptoms
- Most common diagnosis among children complaining of abdominal pain (up to 33% of all cases); extreme care should be taken before diagnosing this disorder in very young or old and immunocompromised patients
- Symptoms and signs: patient appears comfortable; no fever, normal vital signs, no evidence of peritoneal irritation
- Imaging: CT scan is specific in ruling out surgical causes of abdominal pain
- Perform CBC; abdominal or pelvic CT may be indicated; possible admission for 24-hour observation if a surgical cause is contemplated (most commonly "rule out appendicitis"); patients with recurrent abdominal symptoms may need gastroenterology consult

■ Differential Diagnosis

- Surgical cause of abdominal pain: appendicitis, cholecystitis, diverticulitis, gastroenteritis, mesenteric vascular occlusion

■ Treatment

- Avoid narcotics; nonsteroidal anti-inflammatory drugs may be beneficial and are nonaddictive
- Evaluate for other problems

■ Pearl

Beware of patients labeled with nonspecific abdominal pain: they may have real disease.

Reference

Doherty GM, Boey JH: The acute abdomen. In Way LW, Doherty GM (editors): Current Surgical Diagnosis & Treatment, 11th ed. McGraw-Hill, 2003.

Pelvic Inflammatory Disease

- **Essentials of Diagnosis**
  - Also referred to as salpingitis or endometritis; most common in young, nulliparous, sexually active women with multiple partners
  - Symptoms and signs include lower abdominal pain, fever and chills, menstrual disturbances, purulent cervical discharge, cervical and adnexal tenderness, right upper quadrant pain (perihepatitis in Fitz-Hugh and Curtis syndrome)
  - Laboratory tests: endocervical culture for *Neisseria gonorrhoeae* and *Chlamydia trachomatis;* β-hCG
  - Admit the patient for clinical toxicity, tubo-ovarian abscess, or pregnancy

- **Differential Diagnosis**
  - Rule out ectopic pregnancy, septic abortion, torsed or hemorrhagic ovarian cyst
  - Other causes of lower abdominal pain: appendicitis, diverticulitis, gastroenteritis

- **Treatment**
  - Early antibiotic therapy against *N gonorrhoeae, C trachomatis*, and enteric organisms is essential to prevent long-term sequelae
  - Diagnostic laparoscopy used to confirm PID if diagnosis is uncertain or if no clinical response to antibiotics in 48 hours
  - Unilateral adnexectomy for isolated unilateral disease
  - Sexual partner should be examined and treated appropriately
  - Inpatient IV antibiotic regimens: cefoxitin or cefotetan + doxycycline; clindamycin + gentamicin
  - Outpatient antibiotic regimens: single-dose IV cefoxitin or ceftriaxone + doxycycline orally; ofloxacin + metronidazole
  - Prognosis: 25% of women develop long-term sequelae

- **Pearl**

Always do a pelvic examination on women with lower abdominal pain.

Reference

Monif GRG: Pelvic inflammatory disease redefined. Infect Med 2001;18:190.

Porphyria, Acute

- ■ Essentials of Diagnosis
  - Acute porphyrias are a group of inherited diseases that arise from errors in heme biosynthesis, leading to overproduction of a porphyrin species
  - Classic patient is a young woman (teens to early 20s) with an unexplained abdominal crisis; abdominal symptoms are thought to be due to acute (abdominal visceral) autonomic dysfunction
  - Acute porphyria may be precipitated by starvation or certain drugs, classically barbiturates, anticonvulsants, and sulfonamides
  - Symptoms and signs include intermittent abdominal pain varying from mild colic to acute abdomen; fever is absent
  - Laboratory findings: increased amount of porphobilinogen in the urine; freshly voided specimen may turn dark when exposed to bright light and room air
  - Workup: perform CBC, basic blood chemistries, urine porphobilinogen, abdominal pelvic CT scan with IV and oral contrast to rule out surgical cause

- ■ Differential Diagnosis
  - Causes of acute abdomen: appendicitis, diverticulitis, cholecystitis, PID, gastroenteritis

- ■ Treatment
  - IV glucose (≥300 g carbohydrate per day), hematin administration, analgesics, correction of hyponatremia
  - Indications for operation: in confusing cases, diagnostic laparoscopy may exclude an abdominal surgical catastrophe
  - Prognosis: 3-fold increase in mortality in patients recognized to have acute intermittent porphyria

- ■ Pearl

Occasionally, hoofbeats are from unicorns.

Reference

Hambleton J, Toy P: Special medical problems in surgical patients. In Way LW, Doherty GM (editors): Current Surgical Diagnosis & Treatment, 11th ed. McGraw-Hill, 2003.

Pyelonephritis, Acute

- ■ Essentials of Diagnosis
  - Bacterial infection of the upper urinary tract; usually ascending infection; often incompetent ureterovesical junction
  - In men, frequently due to obstructive uropathy; associated with vesicoureteral reflux in children <1 year
  - Symptoms and signs include high fever, chills, dysuria, pyuria
  - Laboratory findings: bacteriuria, leukocytosis, microscopic hematuria, bacteremia
  - Workup: perform CBC, abdominal x-ray; evaluate males for obstruction with ultrasound; perform voiding cystourethrogram in children <1 year

- ■ Differential Diagnosis
  - Acute cystitis, ureteral colic, renal colic, renal infarct
  - Pancreatitis
  - Ruptured abdominal aortic aneurysm
  - Psoas abscess, pelvic abscess, acute salpingitis

- ■ Treatment
  - Nonoperative: IV hydration to ensure good urine production; symptomatic therapy for flank pain and irritative voiding symptoms; empiric antibiotic therapy until culture results available, then specific IV antibiotics; evaluate for obstructive uropathy if no clinical improvement in 48 hours
  - Surgery: indications include obstructive uropathy, perinephric abscess, vesicoureteral reflux; complications include perinephric or psoas abscess, chronic pyelonephritis, acute renal failure, chronic renal insufficiency

- ■ Pearl

Recurrent UTIs in women, and any UTI in men, should prompt an evaluation for reflux or obstruction.

Reference

Williams RD et al: Urology. In Way LW, Doherty GM (editors): Current Surgical Diagnosis & Treatment, 11th ed. McGraw-Hill, 2003.

Ureteral or Renal Calculi

■ Essentials of Diagnosis

- Many affected patients have a history of renal calculi; about 50% chance of second stone within 5 years of first episode
- Symptoms and signs include costovertebral angle or flank pain; pain may radiate to the ipsilateral lower abdominal quadrant; hematuria; nausea, vomiting, intestinal ileus; radiographic evidence of renal or ureteral calculus; fever with proximal infection; nonobstructive calculi are typically asymptomatic
- Hypercalciuria is a metabolic risk factor and occurs in hyperparathyroidism, excess calcium and vitamin D intake, immobilization osteoporosis, Paget disease, sarcoidosis, dehydration; urea-splitting bacteria create magnesium-ammonium phosphate (struvite) stones; metabolic stones form from the hypersecretion of uric acid or cystine
- Laboratory findings: hypercalcemia and hypophosphatemia consistent with hyperparathyroidism; hyperchloremic metabolic acidosis consistent with renal tubular acidosis with secondary renal calcifications
- Spiral CT without contrast can distinguish among stones, tumor, and blood clots; excretory urography verifies stone location and provides information on renal function; spiral CT without contrast ("stone protocol") is best test in urgent setting

■ Differential Diagnosis

- Symptomatic or ruptured abdominal aortic aneurysm
- Proximal infection
- Urologic neoplasm

■ Treatment

- 80% of ureteral stones pass spontaneously
- Extracorporeal shock-wave lithotripsy for renal pelvis calculi
- For most proximal and mid ureteral calculi <1 cm, ureteroscopic treatment with laser or other lithotripsy device
- Metabolic workup for patients with >1 calculus, family history of calculi, recurrent UTIs, or other risk factors
- Prevention: increase fluid intake; combat UTIs; minimize calcium and vitamin D intake for calcium-based stones

■ Pearl

Lack of blood in the urine does not eliminate renal calculus from the differential diagnosis.

References

Ramakumar S et al: Renal calculi: Percutaneous management. Urol Clin North Am 2000;27:617.

Spencer BA et al: Helical CT and ureteral colic. Urol Clin North Am 2000;27:231.

7

Peritoneal Cavity

Endometriosis

- ### Essentials of Diagnosis
    - Deposits of endometrium outside of the uterus that respond to hormonal cycles
    - Prevalence in United States is 2% among fertile women and 3- to 4-fold greater in infertile women
    - Symptoms and signs include dysmenorrhea; constant aching lower abdominal pain, beginning 2–7 days before the onset of menses and increasing in severity until menstrual flow subsides; infertility; dyspareunia
    - Ultrasound often shows complex fluid-filled masses that cannot be distinguished from neoplasms; clinical diagnosis is presumptive and must be confirmed in severe cases

- ### Differential Diagnosis
    - Pelvic inflammatory disease
    - Uterine myomas
    - Ovarian neoplasms, polycystic ovary disease
    - Acute appendicitis
    - Ectopic pregnancy, threatened abortion

- ### Treatment
    - Goal is to ameliorate symptoms and preserve fertility
    - Mainstay of therapy is medical inhibition of ovulation; laparoscopy or laparotomy to resect or ablate lesions, with or without suspension of the uterus for patients <35 years to preserve reproductive function (controversial)
    - Surgery is indicated for failure of medical management
    - Medications: gonadotropin-releasing hormone analogs
    - Prognosis for reproductive function in mild or moderate endometriosis is good with conservative management

- ### Pearl

Always compare the timing of chronic abdominal symptoms to the menstrual cycle.

Reference

Reddy S et al: Treatment of endometriosis. Clin Obstet Gynecol 1998;41:387.

Mesenteric & Omental Cysts

- ■ Essentials of Diagnosis
  - Rare lesions thought to result from sequestration of lymphatic tissue during development
  - Characterized by thin walls lined with endothelial cells without surrounding smooth muscle; cysts may be filled with serous lymphatic fluid (common in the mesocolon and omentum) or chyle (common in small bowel mesentery)
  - Symptoms and signs include bleeding, rupture, torsion, and possible infection of the cyst; soft, mobile abdominal mass; chronic abdominal pain
  - Ultrasound demonstrates a thin-walled, hypoechoic, homogeneous mass that may be uniloculated or multiloculated
  - Computed tomography (CT) scan shows a thin-walled fluid-density mass that may be uniloculated or multiloculated

- ■ Differential Diagnosis
  - Pancreatic pseudocysts
  - Enteric duplication
  - Echinococcal cysts
  - Retroperitoneal tumors
  - Tumor metastasis
  - Large ovarian cysts
  - Pseudomyxoma peritonei

- ■ Treatment
  - Simple excision of the cyst without resection of adjacent organs or major neurovascular structures
  - Partial excision with marsupialization is alternative when complete excision is not possible
  - Internal intestinal drainage is an option, particularly if cyst is adjacent to intestinal wall and may be an enteric duplication
  - Complications: volvulus of cyst with vascular compromise and infarction of the adjacent intestine, bleeding into the cyst, cyst rupture into the abdominal cavity, cyst infection

- ■ Pearl

A broad, ordered differential diagnosis and thorough preoperative assessment can accurately identify this unusual lesion.

Reference

Doherty GM, Boey JH: Peritoneal cavity. In Way LW, Doherty GM (editors): Current Surgical Diagnosis & Treatment, 11th ed. McGraw-Hill, 2003.

Peritoneal Neoplasms

- **Essentials of Diagnosis**
  - Most tumors affecting the peritoneum are secondary implants from intraperitoneal cancers (eg, ovarian, gastric, pancreatic); primary peritoneal tumors are derived from mesodermal lining of the peritoneum
  - History of asbestos exposure in malignant mesothelioma
  - Pseudomyxoma peritonei is usually from a low-grade mucinous cystadenocarcinoma of the appendix or ovary that secretes large amounts of mucus-containing epithelial cells
  - Symptoms and signs include weight loss, crampy abdominal pain, large abdominal mass, or distention due to ascites
  - Perform diagnostic paracentesis for lactic dehydrogenase level, albumin, amylase, triglyceride level, white blood cell count, cytologic studies, Gram stain, and culture
  - Percutaneous biopsy of accessible peritoneal thickening versus diagnostic laparoscopy with biopsy
  - CT scans of lower thorax and abdomen show pleural effusions, ascites, peritoneal and mesenteric thickening

- **Differential Diagnosis**
  - Peritoneal mesotheliomas
  - Well-differentiated papillary mesotheliomas
  - Pseudomyxoma peritonei
  - Benign appendiceal mucocele
  - Adenocarcinomatosis

- **Treatment**
  - Palliative cytoreductive surgery: gross tumor debulking and omentectomy (plus appendectomy and bilateral salpingo-oophorectomy in pseudomyxoma peritonei), intraperitoneal chemotherapy, adjuvant intracavitary radiation, cisplatin- or doxorubicin-based adjuvant chemotherapy for malignant mesothelioma, fluorouracil-based adjuvant chemotherapy for pseudomyxoma peritonei
  - Prognosis: for malignant mesothelioma, long-term survivors (>1 year) have been reported with cytoreductive surgery combined with intraperitoneal chemotherapy; for pseudomyxoma peritonei, survival is 50% at 5 years and 30% at 10 years

- **Pearl**

The combination of tobacco use and asbestos exposure increases the risk of mesothelioma dramatically.

Reference

Sugarbaker PH: Management of peritoneal-surface malignancy: The surgeon's role. Langenbecks Arch Surg 1999;384:576.

Peritonitis, Bacterial

- **Essentials of Diagnosis**
  - A suppurative response of the peritoneal lining to direct bacterial contamination
  - Symptoms and signs include fever and chills, tachycardia, acute abdomen, free air on plain films
  - Primary bacterial peritonitis is caused mainly by hematogenous spread or transluminal invasion in patients with advanced liver disease and reduced ascitic fluid protein concentration
  - Secondary bacterial peritonitis commonly follows disruption of a hollow viscus; physical signs may be subtle in very young, elderly, or immunosuppressed patients
  - Abdominal x-ray shows free air and ileus pattern and may suggest the primary cause
  - Water-soluble contrast study shows location of perforated viscus
  - Abdominal pelvic CT scan with intravenous (IV) and oral contrast is best for finding source of bacterial peritonitis, although operation should not be delayed to obtain this test in patients with an acute abdomen

- **Differential Diagnosis**
  - Appendicitis
  - Perforated gastroduodenal ulcers
  - Diverticulitis
  - Gangrenous cholecystitis
  - Acute salpingitis
  - Nonvascular small bowel perforation
  - Mesenteric ischemia

- **Treatment**
  - Resuscitation with IV fluids and electrolyte replacement
  - Operative control of abdominal sepsis
  - Systemic empiric antibiotics that cover aerobic and anaerobic enteric organisms; directed antibiotic therapy based on operative or aspiration cultures
  - Prognosis: mortality for generalized peritonitis is 40%

- **Pearl**

Appropriate antibiotic coverage and careful monitoring of renal function are key.

Reference

Troidle L et al: Differing outcomes of gram-positive and gram-negative peritonitis. Am J Kidney Dis 1998;32:623.

Retroperitoneal Abscess

■ **Essentials of Diagnosis**

- Primary abscesses are caused by hematogenous bacterial spread, most commonly of *Staphylococcus aureus*
- Secondary abscesses result from spread of infection from adjacent organs, principally the intestine
- Symptoms and signs include fever; flank, abdominal, back, or thigh pain; leukocytosis
- CT scan most accurately delineates these lesions and can differentiate between retroperitoneal hematomas and tumors; abscesses are confined to specific compartments, whereas neoplasms frequently violate fascial barriers
- Perform complete blood count; abdominal or pelvic CT scan with IV and oral contrast is essential

■ **Differential Diagnosis**

- Crohn disease
- Ruptured appendicitis
- Pancreatitis
- Perforated diverticulitis
- Posterior penetrating duodenal ulcer
- Rule out intra-abdominal process with retroperitoneal extension

■ **Treatment**

- Percutaneous drainage may be attempted in well-defined uniloculated abscesses; percutaneous catheter drainage is less successful for retroperitoneal abscesses than for intra-abdominal abscesses
- Most patients require open surgical debridement and drainage, ideally through an extraperitoneal flank approach, and systemic empiric antibiotics that cover aerobic and anaerobic enteric organisms
- Prognosis: retroperitoneal abscesses are difficult to drain completely, so residual or recurrent abscess formation is common; mortality approaches 25%

■ **Pearl**

Consider ureteral stent placement to guide a safe dissection and abscess drainage if open operation is necessary.

Reference

Farthmann EH, Schoffel U: Epidemiology and pathophysiology of intraabdominal infections (IAI). Infection 1998;26:329.

Retroperitoneal Fibrosis

- ■ Essentials of Diagnosis
  - Extensive fibrotic encasement of the retroperitoneal tissues; diffuse desmoplastic involvement of the retroperitoneum may cause obstructive jaundice or small or large bowel obstruction
  - Classic diagnostic triad includes bilateral hydronephrosis/hydroureter, medial deviation of the ureters, extrinsic ureteral compression at the L4–L5 level
  - Ultrasound demonstrates hydronephrosis; CT scan or magnetic resonance imaging shows fibrotic process and the classic diagnostic triad
  - Take complete history including risk factors and symptoms of systemic inflammatory diseases, such as Sjögren syndrome

- ■ Differential Diagnosis
  - Retroperitoneal hematoma, retroperitoneal abscess, retroperitoneal sarcoma, retroperitoneal teratoma
  - Rule out underlying malignancy, most commonly metastatic carcinoma or lymphoma

- ■ Treatment
  - Perform urinary decompression with ureteral stents or percutaneous nephrostomy
  - Repair abdominal aortic aneurysm if present
  - Discontinue suspect medications and initiate anti-inflammatory medications; prednisone and other immunosuppressants have been used with varying success
  - Prognosis: gradual resolution is likely if no underlying cancer

- ■ Pearl

Avoid open operation if possible because fibrosis makes safe dissection difficult.

Reference

Marzano A et al: Treatment of idiopathic retroperitoneal fibrosis using cyclosporine. Ann Rheum Dis 2001;60:427.

Retroperitoneal Hemorrhage

- ■ Essentials of Diagnosis
  - Occurs in patients with a history of trauma; critically ill patients taking anticoagulation or antiplatelet medications; or patients with femoral vascular access, a common cause of clinically silent, large retroperitoneal hematoma
  - Traumatic retroperitoneal hematomas are divided into 3 anatomic zones: zone 1 is centrally located, associated with pancreatico-duodenal injuries or major abdominal vascular injury; zone 2 is in the flank or perinephric region, associated with injuries to the genitourinary system or colon; zone 3 is in the pelvis, associated with pelvic fractures or ileal-femoral vascular injury
  - Symptoms and signs depend on location of retroperitoneal hemorrhage and include femoral nerve palsy; flank and groin ecchymosis is a late sign of retroperitoneal hemorrhage
  - Cardinal laboratory finding is a falling hematocrit; perform serial hematocrit evaluations and assess coagulation
  - CT scan differentiates among hematoma, tumor, and abscess

- ■ Differential Diagnosis
  - Retroperitoneal tumor, retroperitoneal abscess, intraperitoneal process with retroperitoneal extension
  - Rule out associated vascular or adjacent organ injury

- ■ Treatment
  - Obtain large-bore IV access; type and cross 6 U packed red blood cells; normalize coagulation factors
  - Patients with spontaneous retroperitoneal hemorrhage and blunt zone-3 injuries with falling hematocrit should have angiogram with focal embolization
  - Surgery is indicated for all zone-1 injuries, penetrating zone-2 injuries, blunt zone-2 injuries with expanding hematoma, penetrating zone-3 injuries, and evidence of femoral nerve palsy
  - Prognosis: depends on location and severity of injury

- ■ Pearl

Resuscitation and correction of coagulopathy will resolve most cases of spontaneous hemorrhage.

Reference

Sartolli KH et al: Nonoperative management of hepatic, splenic, and renal injuries in adults with multiple injuries. J Trauma 2000;49:56.

8

Hernias

Abdominal Wall Hernias, Noninguinal

- **Essentials of Diagnosis**
  - Typically manifests clinically with an asymptomatic bulge or small bowel obstruction; incarceration and strangulation are common because of the elusive nature of these fascial defects
  - Noninguinal abdominal wall hernias are much less common than inguinal or incisional hernias
  - Symptoms, signs, and hernia sites: spigelian hernia occurs at lateral edge of rectus muscle at level of the umbilicus; lumbodorsal hernia: Grynfeltt occurs at superior lumbar triangle; Petit occurs at inferior lumbar triangle; perineal hernia appears as a reducible perineal bulge

- **Differential Diagnosis**
  - Richter hernia: any strangulated hernia in which only part of the bowel wall becomes ischemic and gangrenous
  - Littre hernia: a hernia that contains Meckel diverticulum in the hernia sac
  - Obturator hernia: herniation through the obturator canal
  - Perineal hernia: myofascial defect of the perineum, usually after perineal surgery
  - Interparietal hernia: hernia between layers of abdominal wall
  - Sciatic hernia: outpouching of intra-abdominal contents through the greater sciatic foramen
  - Traumatic hernia: myofascial defect from direct blunt abdominal injury
  - Supravesicular hernia: myofascial defect adjacent to Cooper's ligament with visceral herniation anterior to urinary bladder

- **Treatment**
  - Uncomplicated abdominal wall defects can be approached electively, typically in outpatient setting
  - Patients with bowel obstruction require resuscitation and urgent operative reduction and repair
  - Prognosis: mortality rate is 13–40% with obturator hernias, making them the most lethal

- **Pearl**

Reduction of painful incarcerated hernia contents can create an intra-abdominal perforation.

References

Naude G et al: Obturator hernia is an unsuspected diagnosis. Am J Surg 1997;174:72.

Thor K: Lumbar hernia. Acta Chir Scand 1985;151:389.

Abdominal Wall Mass

- **Essentials of Diagnosis**
  - Rectus hematomas follow abdominal wall trauma or occur spontaneously in patients receiving anticoagulant therapy
  - Spontaneous abdominal wall metastases are usually associated with lung and pancreatic adenocarcinoma; any intra-abdominal malignancy can extend into the abdominal wall or secondarily seed laparotomy incisions
  - Symptoms and signs: rectus hematoma is an exquisitely tender mass that becomes more painful with flexion of the abdominal wall; surrounding ecchymosis is the classic finding; soft-tissue neoplasms usually are asymptomatic and grow slowly
  - Laboratory findings may include coagulopathy with rectus sheath hematoma; leukocytosis with deep wound infection or abdominal wall abscess
  - Ultrasound differentiates between a solid and a fluid-filled mass; computed tomography (CT) differentiates among hematoma, fat, soft tissue, and fluid-density lesions
  - Workup: obtain careful history and physical examination; perform CT or magnetic resonance imaging when solid mass is suspicious for abdominal wall metastasis, soft-tissue sarcoma, or desmoid tumor; perform percutaneous biopsy for solid mass

- **Differential Diagnosis**
  - Rectus hematoma, deep wound infection, abdominal wall abscess, incisional hernia
  - Tumor metastasis, desmoid tumor, soft-tissue sarcoma

- **Treatment**
  - Rectus sheath hematoma: correct coagulopathy, avoid antiplatelet medications, control pain, and provide expectant management
  - Soft-tissue mass: perform radiography with percutaneous or incisional biopsy
  - Deep wound infection or abdominal wall abscess: perform surgical debridement with serial dressing changes

- **Pearl**

Consider the history of onset carefully to generate an accurate differential diagnosis.

Reference

Doherty GM, Boey JR: The acute abdomen. In Way LW, Doherty GM (editors): Current Surgical Diagnosis & Treatment, 11th ed. McGraw-Hill, 2003.

Femoral Hernia

- **Essentials of Diagnosis**
  - Groin bulge inferior to the inguinal ligament elicited with the Valsalva maneuver
  - Differentiation between inguinal and femoral hernias is difficult clinically and often not appreciated until the hernia sac is dissected free; femoral hernia protrudes through the femoral canal, bordered by the inguinal ligament superiorly, the pubic ramus inferior-medially, and the femoral vein laterally; 1.8:1 female predominance
  - Symptoms and signs usually include asymptomatic inguinal bulge; as hernia enlarges, discomfort may radiate into the ipsilateral thigh or groin
  - Ultrasound, although rarely needed, can verify a femoral hernia sac and differentiate between a hernia and inguinal lymphadenopathy

- **Differential Diagnosis**
  - Inguinal hernia
  - Hydrocele
  - Cord mass
  - Strained groin muscle

- **Treatment**
  - Surgical repair is needed unless there are specific contraindications; both open and laparoscopic repairs are common
  - Immediate surgical repair for incarcerated or strangulated femoral hernia
  - Elective outpatient repair for uncomplicated femoral hernia
  - Prognosis: recurrence rates are <5% in most series

- **Pearl**

Anticipate the difficulty of this diagnosis when discussing femoral "lymph node" biopsy with patients.

Reference

Glassow F: Femoral hernia. Review of 2,105 repairs in a 17 year period. Am J Surg 1985;150:353.

Incisional (Ventral) Hernia

- **Essentials of Diagnosis**
  - Bulge elicited by Valsalva maneuver immediately over or adjacent to a laparotomy incision; the fascial defect progressively increases in size; 11% of all laparotomies result in incisional hernia
  - Symptoms and signs include discomfort or a heavy sensation associated with the hernia bulge; incarcerated hernia is exquisitely painful to palpation and may cause small bowel obstructive symptoms; strangulated hernia may present as acute abdomen
  - Abdominal pelvic CT scan is excellent for detecting incisional hernias and characterizing involved viscera

- **Differential Diagnosis**
  - Diastasis recti
  - Stitch granuloma
  - Epigastric hernia
  - Incisional metastasis

- **Treatment**
  - Minimize or eliminate medications deleterious to wound healing, such as corticosteroids
  - Weight loss in obese patients
  - Incisional hernias should be repaired in all patients without medical contraindications; operative repair can be laparoscopic or open
  - Prognosis: recurrence rate after mesh repair is >20%; recurrence rate after suture repair is >40% for large hernias

- **Pearl**

Weight reduction decreases the symptoms of hernias and recurrence after repair.

Reference

Toy FK et al: Prospective, multicenter study of laparoscopic ventral hernioplasty: Preliminary results. Surg Endosc 1998;12:955.

Inguinal Hernia

- **Essentials of Diagnosis**
  - Groin bulge elicited with the Valsalva maneuver
  - Indirect: patent processus vaginalis extension lateral to the inferior epigastrics in the anterior-medial position of the spermatic cord
  - Direct: developed weakness in the abdominal wall located at Hesselbach triangle (inguinal ligament inferiorly, lateral edge of the rectus medially, and inferior epigastric vessels superior-laterally)
  - Pantaloon hernia: combined direct and indirect inguinal hernia
  - 5–10% of the world population will develop inguinal hernia at some point; nearly all hernias in infants, children, and young adults are indirect
  - Symptoms and signs typically include asymptomatic inguinal bulge; patients may complain of a full or dragging sensation; coughing or straining helps demonstrate small hernias

- **Differential Diagnosis**
  - Femoral hernia
  - Hydrocele
  - Cord mass
  - Strained groin muscle

- **Treatment**
  - Inguinal hernias should be repaired surgically unless there are specific contraindications; both open and laparoscopic approaches are commonly used
  - Complications: strangulated inguinal hernia with visceral necrosis, recurrence
  - Prognosis: recurrence rate is <5% in most series

- **Pearl**

Reduction of painful incarcerated hernia contents can create an intra-abdominal perforation.

Reference

Kark AE et al: 3175 primary inguinal hernia repairs: Advantages of ambulatory open mesh repair using local anesthesia. J Am Coll Surg 1998;186:447.

Umbilical Hernia

- **Essentials of Diagnosis**
    - Bulge elicited by the Valsalva maneuver at the umbilicus; the hernia sac usually contains only pre-peritoneal fat, although small bowel or other abdominal viscera may be present
    - Symptoms and signs typically include asymptomatic umbilical bulge; patients may complain of discomfort, fullness, or heaviness
    - Ultrasound can detect fascial defects and differentiate between an incarcerated umbilical hernia and a solid mass

- **Differential Diagnosis**
    - Epigastric hernia
    - Urachal cyst
    - Primary or metastatic abdominal wall neoplasm

- **Treatment**
    - Minimize or eliminate medications deleterious to wound healing, such as corticosteroids
    - Weight loss in obese patients
    - Control of ascites in cirrhotic patients
    - Surgical repair can be laparoscopic or open
    - Complications: postoperative wound or mesh infection, recurrence

- **Pearl**

Reduction of painful incarcerated hernia contents can create an intra-abdominal perforation.

Reference

Deveney K: Hernias & other lesions of the abdominal wall. In Way LW, Doherty GM (editors): Current Surgical Diagnosis & Treatment, 11th ed. McGraw-Hill, 2003.

Section III

Noncardiac Thoracic Surgery

Chapters

Noncardiac Thoracic Surgery

Bronchial Adenomas & Carcinoid Tumors of Lung

- **Essentials of Diagnosis**
  - Bronchial gland adenomas: 5% of all lung cancer; misnomer because vast majority are malignant
  - Carcinoid lung tumors: 85% of bronchial adenomas; classified as typical or atypical; derived from Kulchitsky cells; located in central, proximal airways; slow growing; can metastasize widely, rarely cause carcinoid syndrome
  - Adenoid cystic carcinoma (cylindromas): locally aggressive; metastases involve lung; slow growing; amenable to resection
  - Mucoepidermoid cancer: rare tumor; mucus-secreting cells and squamous cells present
  - Mucous gland adenomas: truly benign

- **Differential Diagnosis**
  - More common types of pulmonary malignancy
  - Infections

- **Treatment**
  - Resection is primary treatment; lobectomy or sleeve
  - Adenoid cystic carcinomas: require generous margins and frozen section examination at surgery
  - Prognosis: very good in general; lymph node and distant metastases portend poor prognosis

- **Pearl**

The prognosis for bronchial adenomas is better than for most pulmonary malignancies.

Reference

Gould MK et al: Accuracy of positron emission tomography for diagnosis of pulmonary nodules and mass lesions: A meta-analysis. JAMA 2001;285:914.

Bronchiectasis

- **Essentials of Diagnosis**
  - Clinical syndrome marked by chronic dilation of bronchi, paroxysmal cough producing mucopurulent sputum, recurrent pulmonary infections
  - Two main types: saccular follows most infections and bronchial obstruction; cylindric is associated with post-tuberculosis (TB) bronchiectasis
  - Symptoms and signs include recurrent febrile episodes, chronic or intermittent cough producing foul-smelling sputum (up to 500 mL/d), hemoptysis (about 50% of patients)

- **Differential Diagnosis**
  - Congenital diseases: Kartagener syndrome, cystic fibrosis, Williams-Campbell syndrome, Mounier-Kuhn syndrome
  - Immunoglobulin deficiency; α_1-antitrypsin deficiency
  - Obstruction from neoplasm or foreign body

- **Treatment**
  - In most cases, conservative medical treatment is sufficient
  - Surgery: goals are to remove all active disease, preserve functioning lung as much as possible
  - Surgery is indicated for localized, completely resectable disease or significant symptoms despite medical treatment in patients with adequate pulmonary reserve
  - Prognosis: local disease has 80% success with surgery; diffuse disease has 36% surgical success
  - Prevention: long-term antibiotic therapy for suppression

- **Pearl**

Pulmonary hygiene is important to maintain the best possible function.

Reference

Ip M et al: Multivariate analysis of factors affecting pulmonary function in bronchiectasis. Respiration 1993;60:45.

Broncholithiasis

- Essentials of Diagnosis
  - Causes include calcified parabronchial lymph node eroding into bronchial wall lumen (most common); severely inspissated mucus may calcify
  - Broncholiths may remain attached to bronchial wall, lodge in bronchus, or be expectorated (lithoptysis)
  - Diagnosis is confirmed by lithoptysis or presence of broncholith
  - Symptoms and signs include hemoptysis; lithoptysis (30%); cough, sputum production, pleuritic chest pain; fever, chills; wheezing; pneumonia from obstructive broncholith

- Differential Diagnosis
  - Other causes of hemoptysis (pneumonia, tumor, trauma)
  - Aspirated foreign body

- Treatment
  - Treat underlying pulmonary disease and remove stone
  - Bronchoscopy is successful 20% of time to remove stone
  - Surgery is required 80% of time; bronchotomy and stone extraction or segmentectomy/lobectomy
  - Prognosis: excellent after surgery

- Pearl

Treatment of the underlying cause of stone formation is important.

Reference

Galdermans D et al: Broncholithiasis: Present clinical spectrum. Respir Med 1990;84:155.

Chest Wall Osteomyelitis

- ■ Essentials of Diagnosis
  - Sternal infections are common after median sternotomy; increased risk among diabetic patients in whom bilateral internal mammary arteries have been used for coronary revascularization
  - Symptoms and signs include postoperative wound infection or mediastinitis in sternum; erythema, fever, fluctuance

- ■ Differential Diagnosis
  - Costal cartilage infection
  - Bone tumor
  - Cartilage tumor
  - Tietze syndrome
  - Chest wall metastasis
  - Eroding aortic aneurysm
  - Bronchocutaneous fistula

- ■ Treatment
  - Surgery is indicated for deep infection; perform aggressive debridement with cultures and muscle flap closure
  - Medications: intravenous (IV) antibiotics

- ■ Pearl

Prevention of surgical site infection is far preferable to treatment of infection.

Reference

Siegman-Igra Y et al: Serious infectious complications of midsternotomy: A review of bacteriology and antimicrobial therapy. Scand J Infect Dis 1990;22:633.

Chest Wall Tumors, Benign Skeletal

- ■ Essentials of Diagnosis
  - Fibrous dysplasia: accounts for 33% of benign skeletal tumors; usually single tumor; associated with trauma
  - Chondromas, osteochondromas, myxochondromas: together equal 30–45% of benign skeletal tumors
  - Eosinophilic granuloma: benign form of Letterer-Siwe disease or Hand-Schüller-Christian disease
  - Hemangioma: cavernous hemangioma of ribs is painful mass during childhood
  - Symptoms and signs: most often painless
  - Workup: perform computed tomography (CT) scan of thorax including bone windows; bone scan; incisional biopsy for large mass (>4 cm)

- ■ Differential Diagnosis
  - Can be difficult to distinguish from malignant lesions

- ■ Treatment
  - Wide local excision often necessary for cure

- ■ Pearl

Diagnostic biopsy must be planned to facilitate definitive resection.

Reference

Burt M et al: Primary bony and cartilaginous sarcomas of chest wall: Results of therapy. Ann Thorac Surg 1992;54:226.

Chest Wall Tumors, Benign Soft Tissue

- **Essentials of Diagnosis**
  - Lipomas: most common benign tumors
  - Neurogenic tumors: arise from intercostal nerves; solitary neurofibromas most common
  - Cavernous hemangiomas: usually painful; occur in children
  - Lymphangiomas: rare lesions seen in children; poorly defined borders
  - Ultrasound and CT scan may aid in diagnosis

- **Differential Diagnosis**
  - Rule out malignant neoplasm

- **Treatment**
  - Surgery is indicated for growing tumors
  - If tumor is large (>5 cm), consider incisional biopsy to rule out malignancy

- **Pearl**

Diagnostic biopsy must be planned to facilitate definitive resection.

Reference

Kim JY et al: Atypical benign lipomatous tumors in the soft tissue. J Comp Assist Tomogr 2002;26:1063.

Chest Wall Tumors, Malignant Skeletal

- ■ Essentials of Diagnosis
  - Chondrosarcoma: most common primary malignancy of chest wall (30%)
  - Osteosarcoma: worse prognosis than chondrosarcoma; propensity to metastasize to lung or bone
  - Myeloma: rare lesion, causing 5–20% of chest wall tumors
  - Ewing sarcoma: 10–15% of primary chest wall tumors
  - Metastatic tumors: kidney, thyroid, lung, breast, prostate, stomach, uterus, or colon; renal and thyroid have high propensity to metastasize to sternum
  - Workup: perform chest film, chest CT scan; incisional or excisional biopsy depending on size and configuration

- ■ Differential Diagnosis
  - Rule out aortic aneurysm before obtaining biopsy specimen of any lesion, especially if pulsatile

- ■ Treatment
  - Surgery is indicated for localized tumor
  - Prognosis: depends on tumor
  - Chondrosarcoma: positive margins give much worse prognosis; histologic grade is clear predictor; for low grade, 5-year survival is 60–80%; for high grade, 25%
  - Osteosarcoma: 5-year survival is 15%; metastases develop in 60–70% of patients after resection
  - Myeloma: 5-year survival is 35–40%; 10-year survival is 15–20%
  - Ewing sarcoma: distant metastasis is common; 5-year survival is 15–48%

- ■ Pearl

Diagnostic biopsy must be planned to facilitate definitive resection.

Reference

Burt M: Primary malignant tumors of the chest wall. The Memorial Sloan-Kettering Cancer Center experience. Chest Surg Clin N Am 1994;4:137.

Chest Wall Tumors, Malignant Soft Tissue

- **Essentials of Diagnosis**
  - Desmoid tumor: low grade
  - Fibrosarcoma: most common in this location, especially in young adults
  - Liposarcoma: 33% of all primary cancers of chest wall, especially in men
  - Neurofibrosarcoma: 2 times more common in this location than any other, often seen in Recklinghausen disease; originates from intercostal nerves
  - Workup: perform chest film, chest CT scan; incisional or excisional biopsy depending on size and configuration

- **Differential Diagnosis**
  - Rule out metastatic disease with chest CT

- **Treatment**
  - Goal is to achieve negative margins (1–2 cm); methylmethacrylate to correct chest wall deformity; soft tissue flaps for coverage
  - Radiation therapy for positive margins; adjuvant chemotherapy if high grade
  - Surgery is indicated for resectable lesion, localized metastatic disease to lung if amenable to negative margins
  - Prognosis: depends on histologic grade; 5-year survival for low grade is 90%, for high grade is 20–50%

- **Pearl**

Diagnostic biopsy incision must be planned to facilitate inclusion in definitive resection.

Reference

Burt M: Primary malignant tumors of the chest wall. The Memorial Sloan-Kettering Cancer Center experience. Chest Surg Clin N Am 1994;4:137.

Empyema

- ■ Essentials of Diagnosis
  - Pyothorax: pus in pleural cavity; usually thick, creamy, malodorous; occurs in setting of pneumonia, lung abscess, bronchiectasis
  - Types include parapneumonic (60%), postsurgical (20%), posttraumatic (10%)
  - Three temporal phases: acute exudative: sterile low-viscosity pleural fluid; transitional (fibrinopurulent): increase in turbidity, white blood cell count, and lactate dehydrogenase; chronic organizing: occurs 7–28 days after disease onset; exudate thickens, causing further fixation of lung
  - Symptoms and signs: rarely asymptomatic; usually causes fever, pleuritic chest pain, dyspnea, hemoptysis, cough, tachycardia, anemia, tachypnea, diminished breath sounds, clubbing
  - Chest film and chest CT show pneumonia, lung abscess, pleural effusion, mediastinal shift away if large empyema

- ■ Differential Diagnosis
  - Pneumonia
  - Pleural effusion
  - Tumor
  - Other sources of infection

- ■ Treatment
  - Goals are to control infection, remove purulent material with lung reexpansion, eliminate underlying disease
  - Pus found on thoracentesis: place chest tube; convert to open drainage; perform sonogram: if no cavity, withdraw tube; if small cavity, evaluate how well it is drained; if large cavity and well drained, slowly advance tube
  - Residual space and continued sepsis: consider open drainage procedures, rib resection; Eloesser procedure: simple rib resection and open flap drainage
  - Monitor treatment with chest CT after chest tube insertion to evaluate adequacy of drainage and lung reexpansion

- ■ Pearl

Drainage of fluid collection and lung reexpansion are critical for resolution of infection.

Reference

Alfageme I et al: Empyema of the thorax in adults: Etiology, microbiologic findings, and management. Chest 1993;103:839.

Lung Abscess

- ■ Essentials of Diagnosis
  - Primary: aspiration of oropharyngeal contents; acute necrotizing pneumonia (*Staphylococcus, Klebsiella*)
  - Secondary: bronchial obstruction (cancer, foreign body); cavitating pulmonary lesions (cancer)
  - Symptoms and signs include cough, fever, dyspnea, pleuritic chest pain; malaise, weight loss if chronic
  - Chest film shows area of intense consolidation or rounded density, with or without air-fluid level; CT scan is helpful in cases of suspected bronchial obstruction

- ■ Differential Diagnosis
  - Primary structural diseases of lungs
  - Cancer

- ■ Treatment
  - Antibiotics are mainstay of treatment; penicillin and clindamycin commonly used; continue antibiotics until complete resolution (3–6 months)
  - Percutaneous drainage if accessible
  - Surgery is indicated for poor response to medical regimen, and possibly percutaneous drainage if accessible; tense abscess (eg, mediastinal shift, shift of diaphragm); evidence of contralateral lung contamination
  - Prognosis: percutaneous drainage results in 1.5% mortality, 10% morbidity; overall mortality rate is 5–20%; medical therapy success is 75–88%; operative patients are cured 90% of time, with 1% mortality; mortality in immunocompromised patients is 28%

- ■ Pearl

Evaluate for underlying pulmonary disease that may precipitate infection.

Reference

Bartlett JG: Antibiotics in lung abscess. Semin Respir Infect 1991;6:103.

Lung Cancer, Primary

- ■ Essentials of Diagnosis
    - Non-small cell lung carcinoma (NSCLC): mostly squamous and adenocarcinoma; 80% of all lung cancers; early without mediastinal involvement is stage I/II; locally advanced is stage IIIA/B; metastatic is stage IV
    - Squamous cell carcinoma: frequent association with tobacco smoking; keratinization; frequently proximal bronchus
    - Adenocarcinoma: most common NSCLC; frequency increasing; subtypes are acinar, papillary, bronchoalveolar, mucus secreting
    - Large cell carcinoma: uncommon
    - Small cell (oat cell) carcinoma: 15% of cases
    - Symptoms and signs: central tumors cause cough, hemoptysis, respiratory distress, pain, pneumonia; peripheral tumors cause cough, chest wall pain, pleural effusions, pulmonary abscess, Horner syndrome, Pancoast syndrome
    - Classic paraneoplastic syndromes: small cell: Eaton-Lambert (myasthenia), syndrome of inappropriate antidiuretic hormone, adrenocorticotropic hormone, carcinoid; squamous cell carcinoma: hypercalcemia; adenocarcinoma: acanthosis nigricans
    - Perform chest CT scan for evaluation of infiltrate, nodule; brain CT scan if neurologic symptoms; positron emission tomography (PET) scan may be important staging test; thoracentesis if pleural effusion to rule out malignancy

- ■ Differential Diagnosis
    - Rule out metastatic disease with imaging and thoracentesis

- ■ Treatment
    - NSCLC: stages I-IIIA are resectable; stages IIIB/IV are often unresectable; for early disease, goal is complete resection; for advanced disease, preoperative chemoradiotherapy
    - Small cell carcinoma: typically chemoradiotherapy
    - Prognosis: NSCLC 5-year survival: stage I, 43–64%; stage II, 30%; stage IIIA, 15–25%; stage IIIB, 5–7%; stage IV, <2%
    - Small cell carcinoma: limited disease 2-year survival: 5–25%; extensive disease 2-year survival: 1–3%

- ■ Pearl

Small cell lung cancer is a poorly differentiated disease that behaves as a systemic illness, even when localized.

References

Friedel G et al: Neoadjuvant chemoradiotherapy of stage III non-small cell lung cancer. Lung Cancer 2000;30:175.

National Comprehensive Cancer Network: Practice Guidelines. http://www.nccn.org

Lung Infection, Aspergillosis

- **Essentials of Diagnosis**
  - Allergic bronchopulmonary aspergillosis: occurs in patients with asthma or cystic fibrosis; fungal growth leads to dilated airways filled with mucus and fungus
  - Invasive aspergillosis: found only in immunocompromised patients
  - Aspergilloma (fungus balls): divided into 2 types: simple, thin-walled cysts with ciliated epithelium surrounded by normal lung; and complex cavities with abnormal surrounding lung tissue
  - Second most common opportunistic fungal infection after candidiasis
  - Symptoms and signs: allergic bronchopulmonary aspergillosis causes cough, fever, wheezing, dyspnea, pleuritic pain, hemoptysis; invasive aspergillosis causes cough, dyspnea, wheezing, aspergilloma

- **Differential Diagnosis**
  - Definitive diagnosis requires demonstration of hyphal tissue invasion or documentation of hyphae on silver stain in suspected aspergilloma

- **Treatment**
  - Allergic bronchopulmonary aspergillosis: medical therapy (corticosteroids)
  - Invasive aspergillosis: amphotericin B
  - Surgery is indicated for hemoptysis secondary to aspergilloma; cavitation secondary to invasive aspergillosis
  - Prognosis: mortality rate is 90% in invasive aspergillosis

- **Pearl**

Invasive disease is common only in immunocompromised hosts and is associated with a high mortality rate.

Reference

Johnson P, Sarosi G: Current therapy of major fungal diseases of the lung. Infect Dis Clin North Am 1991;5:635.

Lung Infection, Blastomycosis

- ■ Essentials of Diagnosis
  - Predilection for upper lobes; hilar mediastinal adenopathy is unusual (unlike in histoplasmosis and coccidioidomycosis)
  - *Blastomycosis dermatitidis* is found in warm, wet, nitrogen-rich soil in east, Midwest, and south (except Florida and New England)
  - Characteristically occurs in males (10:1 male to female ratio) aged 30–60 years; risk factors include poor hygiene, poor housing
  - Symptoms and signs: asymptomatic or flulike symptoms (cough, weight loss, pleuritic pain, fever, hemoptysis, erythema nodosum)
  - Chest film shows pulmonary masses that may mimic malignancy

- ■ Differential Diagnosis
  - Yeast form is found in sputum (33%), bronchoalveolar lavage (38%), biopsy (21%), fine-needle aspiration (7%)

- ■ Treatment
  - No treatment needed if limited disease and asymptomatic
  - Antifungal agents are first-line therapy
  - Medications: nonmeningeal disease: itraconazole for 3 months (>80% response); meningeal disease or failed therapy: amphotericin B

- ■ Pearl

Blastomycosis is usually a limited disease requiring no therapy.

Reference

Johnson P, Sarosi G: Current therapy of major fungal diseases of the lung. Infect Dis Clin North Am 1991;5:635.

Lung Infection, Coccidioidomycosis

- ■ Essentials of Diagnosis
  - • Persistent infection 6–8 weeks after primary; classified into 5 types: persistent pneumonia, chronic progressive pneumonia, miliary coccidioidomycosis, coccidioidal nodules, pulmonary cavities
  - • *Coccidioides immitis* is endemic to Sonoran life zone (Utah, California, Arizona, Nevada, New Mexico), associated with creosote brush; dry heat with brief intense rain essential for fungus; spread by strong winds; in endemic areas, 30–50% of all pulmonary nodules are coccidioidomas
  - • Symptoms and signs: primary infection is asymptomatic in 60%; "desert fever" causes fever, productive cough, pleuritic chest pain, pneumonitis, rash; "desert rheumatism" consists of desert fever with arthralgias; miliary coccidioidomycosis occurs early and rapidly with bilateral diffuse infiltrates

- ■ Differential Diagnosis
  - • Histoplasmosis
  - • TB

- ■ Treatment
  - • For persistent illness or risk of dissemination, treat with antifungal agents
  - • Medications: amphotericin B is standard treatment; fluconazole, ketoconazole, itraconazole for long-term maintenance
  - • Complications: 25–50% of patients requiring antifungal agents relapse
  - • Prognosis: mortality for disseminated and miliary coccidioidomycosis is 50%

- ■ Pearl

Coccidioidomycosis can be dangerous in immunocompromised individuals.

Reference

Johnson P, Sarosi G: Current therapy of major fungal diseases of the lung. Infect Dis Clin North Am 1991;5:635.

Lung Infection, Cryptococcosis

- **Essentials of Diagnosis**
  - Pulmonary fungal infections are rising because of widespread use of broad-spectrum antibiotics, immunosuppressive drugs, and human immunodeficiency virus (HIV) infection
  - *Cryptococcus neoformans*: found in pigeon excreta, grasses, trees, plants, fruits, insects, birds, dairy products; exists also on skin and in nasopharynx, gastrointestinal tract, vagina
  - Symptoms and signs: pulmonary infection may cause cough, pleuritic chest pain, fever; central nervous system infection usually follows asymptomatic pulmonary infection
  - Laboratory findings demonstrate elevated serum antigen (on complement fixation tests)

- **Differential Diagnosis**
  - Histoplasmosis
  - TB

- **Treatment**
  - Medical therapy is warranted in most cases of pulmonary infection even if asymptomatic
  - Surgical resection rarely necessary; open lung biopsy if diagnosis is equivocal
  - Medications: amphotericin B combined with flucytosine; fluconazole and itraconazole for long-term maintenance

- **Pearl**

Cryptococcosis can be dangerous in an immunocompromised host.

Reference

Johnson P, Sarosi G: Current therapy of major fungal diseases of the lung. Infect Dis Clin North Am 1991;5:635.

Lung Infection, Histoplasmosis

- ■ Essentials of Diagnosis
  - Acute infection: flulike syndrome limited to lungs; diffuse nodular disease
  - Chronic infection: several presentations: asymptomatic solitary nodule <3 cm with central calcifications in lower lobes (histoplasmoma); mediastinal granulomas resulting in broncholithiasis, esophageal traction diverticula, superior vena cava (SVC) compression, transesophageal fistulas; fibrosing mediastinitis with SVC, tracheal, or esophageal compression
  - *Histoplasma capsulatum* found in fowl and bat excreta, pigeon roosts, chicken houses, caves, hollow trees, attics, and lofts; endemic to fertile river valleys, such as Mississippi, Missouri, and Ohio Rivers
  - Symptoms and signs include cough, malaise, hemoptysis, fever, weight loss (30% have coexistent TB), solitary pulmonary nodules (15–20% are from histoplasmosis)

- ■ Differential Diagnosis
  - Other causes of pulmonary nodules
  - Other causes of mediastinal adenopathy

- ■ Treatment
  - Medical therapy is indicated in immunocompromised hosts or in cavitary or severe disease
  - Surgery is indicated only for complications
  - Medications: ketoconazole or itraconazole (6 months) for cavitary disease

- ■ Pearl

Fluorodeoxyglucose PET scan may be helpful to distinguish pulmonary histoplasmosis from primary pulmonary tumor.

Reference

Johnson P, Sarosi G: Current therapy of major fungal diseases of the lung. Infect Dis Clin North Am 1991;5:635.

Lung Infection, Mucormycosis

- ■ Essentials of Diagnosis
  - Distinct clinical syndromes: rhinocerebral infection involves direct extension into central nervous system from paranasal sinus infection; cutaneous infection occurs in burn patients; gastrointestinal infection occurs in children with protein-calorie malnutrition; disseminated infection occurs in uremic patients receiving deferoxamine therapy
  - Pulmonary fungal infections are rising because of widespread use of broad-spectrum antibiotics, immunosuppressive drugs, and HIV infection
  - Includes *Rhizopus arrhizus* (most common), *Absidia* species, *Rhizomucor* species; common in decaying fruit, vegetables, soil, and manure; infection occurs in patients with diabetes, leukemia, immunosuppression
  - Symptoms and signs of pulmonary infection include fever, cough, pleuritic chest pain, hemoptysis

- ■ Differential Diagnosis
  - Other chronic pulmonary infections
  - Tumors

- ■ Treatment
  - Amphotericin B is standard treatment
  - Prognosis: mortality is 90% despite best treatment; death is due to fungal sepsis, pulmonary dysfunction, hemoptysis

- ■ Pearl

Necrotic tissue or sequestration of infection can make resolution difficult.

Reference

Johnson P, Sarosi G: Current therapy of major fungal diseases of the lung. Infect Dis Clin North Am 1991;5:635.

Lung Lesions, Metastatic

■ Essentials of Diagnosis

- Pulmonary metastases occur via hematogenous spread from primary site; lymphatic and transbronchial spread are rare; 30% of patients with malignancies develop pulmonary metastases
- Symptoms and signs: most patients are asymptomatic or have cough, hemoptysis, fever, dyspnea, pain

■ Differential Diagnosis

- Second primary tumor
- Pulmonary infection

■ Treatment

- If complete resection cannot resolve all known disease, resection should not be offered
- Surgery: wedge resection is treatment of choice
- Surgery is indicated if primary tumor is controlled or imminently controllable, no other sites of disease, no other therapy can offer comparable results, low operative risk
- Prognosis: best prognosis is for testicular: 51% 5-year survival for all patients; head and neck cancers: 47% 5-year survival; osteogenic or soft tissue sarcomas, renal cell, or colon: 20–35% survival; melanoma: 10–15% survival; rectal cancer with isolated pulmonary metastasis: 55% 5–year survival
- Poor prognosis: multiple or bilateral lesions, >4 lesions on CT, tumor doubling time <40 days, short disease-free interval, advanced age

■ Pearl

Metastasectomy is reasonable only if primary disease is controlled and all disease can be removed.

References

National Comprehensive Cancer Network: Practice Guidelines. http://www.nccn.org
Pogrebniak HW, Pass HI: Initial and reoperative pulmonary metastasectomy: Indications, technique, and results. Semin Surg Oncol 1993;9:142.

Lung Neoplasms, Benign

- **Essentials of Diagnosis**
  - Uncommon; represent <1% of pulmonary tumors
  - Types include fibromas, leiomyomas, neurofibromas, myoblastomas, benign metastasizing leiomyomas
  - Most lesions are peripheral
  - Symptoms and signs: peripheral lesions are asymptomatic; central lesions produce cough, wheezing, hemoptysis, recurrent pneumonia

- **Differential Diagnosis**
  - May be difficult to distinguish from malignant lesions; excision may be necessary for diagnosis

- **Treatment**
  - Wedge resection
  - Surgery is indicated for tissue diagnosis if not obtainable by bronchoscopy
  - Prognosis: excellent

- **Pearl**

Fluorodeoxyglucose PET scan may be helpful to differentiate benign from malignant pulmonary nodules.

Reference

Gould MK et al: Accuracy of positron emission tomography for diagnosis of pulmonary nodules and mass lesions: A meta-analysis. JAMA 2001;285:914.

Mediastinal Masses

- **Essentials of Diagnosis**
  - Divided into 3 regions: anterior, middle (great vessels, heart, trachea, and esophagus), and posterior
  - Neurogenic tumor: posterior mediastinum, often superiorly from intercostal or sympathetic nerves; nerve sheath tumors (eg, schwannoma, neurofibroma) most common (40–65%); usually benign, 10% malignant; may be multiple or dumbbell shaped
  - Mediastinal cystic lesion: arises from pericardium, bronchi, esophagus, or thymus; 75% located near cardiophrenic angles, 75% on right side; 10% are diverticula of pericardial sac that communicate with pericardial space
  - Germ cell tumor: anterior mediastinum; both solid and cystic, may contain teeth or hair; most are metastatic from retroperitoneal disease; <5% are primary tumors; seminoma (40%), embryonal carcinomas and nongestational choriocarcinomas (20%), yolk sac (20%), and teratomas (20%) can have both benign and malignant components
  - Lymphoma: usually disseminated disease; anterior compartment most common but can be anywhere in mediastinum
  - Symptoms and signs: 50% of patients have cough, wheezing, dyspnea, or recurrent pneumonias; hemoptysis, chest pain, weight loss, and dysphagia less common, each in 10% of patients
  - Chest CT is diagnostic test of choice

- **Differential Diagnosis**
  - Lymph node lesions
  - Lung tumors

- **Treatment**
  - Complete resection is treatment of choice, often needed for diagnosis; excisional biopsy preferred to prevent cancer dispersion; perform mediastinoscopy or biopsy cautiously for potentially curable lesions
  - Median sternotomy for anterior masses
  - Thoracotomy for middle and posterior masses
  - Prognosis: nonseminomatous germ cell tumor has 50% 5-year survival; seminoma has 90% 5-year survival; other malignant lesions have <50% cure rate

- **Pearl**

Avoid needle biopsy of lesions that are potentially curable by resection.

References

Gould MK et al: Accuracy of positron emission tomography for diagnosis of pulmonary nodules and mass lesions: A meta-analysis. JAMA 2001;285:914.

National Comprehensive Cancer Network: Practice Guidelines. http://www.nccn.org

Mediastinitis

- **Essentials of Diagnosis**
  - Four primary sources: direct contamination, hematogenous or lymphatic spread (granulomatous), extension of infection from neck or retroperitoneum, extension from lung or pleura
  - Secondary causes include oral surgery, trauma to pharynx, tracheostomy, mediastinoscopy, thyroidectomy
  - Esophageal perforation caused by Boerhaave syndrome, iatrogenic trauma (eg, dilation, esophagogastroduodenoscopy), external trauma, cuffed endotracheal tubes, ingestion of corrosives, carcinoma
  - Symptoms and signs include history of vomiting; severe boring pain in substernal, left or right chest, or epigastric regions, with radiation to back
  - Chest CT, with oral and IV contrast, may help determine level of perforation, degree of soilage, and underlying pathology

- **Differential Diagnosis**
  - Myocardial infarction
  - Esophageal perforation
  - Other causes of chest pain

- **Treatment**
  - Underlying cause determines treatment
  - Initial management: immediate drainage of pleural contamination with chest tube; broad-spectrum antibiotics with fluid hydration
  - Surgery: right thoracotomy gives best access to most of intrathoracic esophagus (including distal portion); iatrogenic perforation <24 hours: 2-layer closure (mucosal layer with interrupted absorbable sutures and muscle closure); perforation >48 hours: wide drainage, resection of esophagus
  - Medications: broad-spectrum antibiotics (including aminoglycosides)
  - Prognosis: 30–60% mortality with esophageal perforation

- **Pearl**

Infection must be drained, ongoing contamination stopped, and adequate antibiotic coverage started, all quickly, to resolve mediastinitis.

Reference

Marty-Ane CH et al: Descending necrotizing mediastinitis. Advantage of mediastinal drainage with thoracotomy. J Thorac Cardiovasc Surg 1994;57:55.

Middle Lobe Syndrome

- **Essentials of Diagnosis**
  - Relapsing lateral pneumonia of right middle pulmonary lobe caused by intermittent obstruction; obstruction most often extrinsic; consider diagnosis with repeated right-sided pneumonia
  - May be caused by compression or erosion of bronchus by adjacent diseased lymph nodes; poor natural drainage and lack of collateral ventilation explain frequency of involvement of right middle lobe

- **Differential Diagnosis**
  - Rule out other causes of obstruction (neoplasm, foreign body)

- **Treatment**
  - Intensive medical therapy is usually adequate
  - Surgery is lobectomy of right middle lobe
  - Surgery is indicated for bronchiectasis, fibrosis of right middle lobe, right middle lobe abscess, intractable recurrent pneumonia, suspicion of neoplasm

- **Pearl**

Always evaluate for an underlying cause of the recurrent pneumonia.

Reference

Ring-Mrozik E et al: Clinical findings in middle lobe syndrome and other processes of pulmonary shrinkage in children (atelectasis syndrome). Eur J Pediatr Surg 1991;1:266.

Pleural Effusion

- **Essentials of Diagnosis**
  - Presence of fluid in pleural space; causes include increased pulmonary hydrostatic pressure, decreased intravascular oncotic pressure, increased capillary permeability, decreased intrapleural pressure (atelectasis), decreased lymphatic drainage (carcinomatosis), rupture of vascular or lymphatic structure (trauma)
  - When nature of fluid is known, more specific terms are used: pyothorax is pus in pleural cavity (empyema); hemothorax is blood in thorax; chylothorax is chyle in thorax; hydrothorax is collection of serous fluid (transudative or exudative)
  - Symptoms and signs include decreased respiratory excursions, diminished breath sounds, dullness to percussion
  - On chest film, blunting of costophrenic angle seen as 250–500 mL of fluid; entire hemithorax effusion evident as >2 L

- **Differential Diagnosis**
  - TB
  - Cancer
  - Congestive heart failure
  - Pneumonia
  - Rheumatoid arthritis or collagen disease
  - Pulmonary embolism

- **Treatment**
  - Malignant effusion: goal is palliation plus lung reexpansion, chest tube, chemical pleurodesis
  - Congestive heart failure: treat underlying failure, diuresis
  - Chylothorax: closed chest tube drainage, low-fat diet, video-assisted thoracoscopic technique: ligation of thoracic duct at diaphragm between aorta and azygous vein
  - Prognosis: varies with underlying cause

- **Pearl**

Thoracentesis to assess fluid is important in the diagnosis of pleural effusion.

Reference

Therapy of pleural effusion: A statement by the Committee on Therapy of the American Thoracic Society. Am Rev Respir Dis 1968;97:479.

Pleural Tumors

- ■ **Essentials of Diagnosis**
  - • Localized fibrous tumor of pleura: previously called "localized mesothelioma"; arises from subpleural fibroblasts; involvement of visceral pleura more common than parietal
  - • Diffuse malignant pleural mesothelioma: most common primary tumor of pleura; strong link to asbestos exposure, with 300 times increased risk; amphibole fibers (eg, crocidolite, amosite) and soil silicate zeolite lodge in terminal airways and migrate to pleura; latency after asbestos exposure is 15–50 years; risk greatly increased by tobacco use
  - • Fine-needle aspiration usually inadequate; biopsy through small incision or video-assisted thoracoscopic surgery

- ■ **Differential Diagnosis**
  - • Pleural effusion
  - • Pulmonary mass or tumor
  - • Pneumonia

- ■ **Treatment**
  - • Localized fibrous tumor of pleura: complete resection; lobectomy usually not required; wedge resection recommended if visceral pleura involved
  - • Diffuse malignant pleural mesothelioma: surgical approach is radical pleuropneumonectomy or parietal pleurectomy with decortication
  - • Chemotherapy, photodynamic therapy, immunotherapy, gene therapy, intraoperative chemoradiation therapy are done at some centers under clinical trials
  - • Prognosis: localized fibrous tumor of pleura has good outcome if resection is complete; diffuse malignant pleural mesothelioma has median survival of 7–16 months

- ■ **Pearl**

The risk of mesothelioma after asbestos exposure is greatly increased by concomitant smoking.

References

Cheng AY: Neoplasms in the mediastinum, chest wall, and pleura. Curr Opin Oncol 1999;6:17.

National Comprehensive Cancer Network: Practice Guidelines. http://www.nccn.org

Pneumonia

- ■ **Essentials of Diagnosis**
  - Represents 13–18% of all nosocomial infections; 25% of patients in intensive care unit develop pneumonia
  - Risk factors include old age, mechanical ventilation, head injury, H_2-receptor blockers or proton pump inhibitors, frequent ventilator setting changes, winter months, large-volume aspiration of gastric contents, thoracic surgery, chronic lung disease
  - Symptoms and signs include fever, increase and change in character of sputum, hypoxia
  - Chest film or CT scan shows pulmonary infiltrate

- ■ **Differential Diagnosis**
  - Atelectasis
  - Pulmonary embolus
  - Other likely causes of fever in clinical situation
  - Lung tumor

- ■ **Treatment**
  - Consider prior antibiotic exposure when choosing therapy; empiric coverage must be appropriate for patient and endogenous flora
  - Respiratory therapy is essential to help patient clear secretions
  - Prognosis: associated mortality is 20–50%; excess risk of death, 33%
  - Prevention: avoid supine position; extubate promptly; give vigorous respiratory therapy; encourage early ambulation to preserve pulmonary clearance mechanisms

- ■ **Pearl**

Prevention of nosocomial pneumonia is preferable to treatment.

Reference

Montravers P et al: Diagnostic and therapeutic management of nosocomial pneumonia in surgical patients: Results of the Eole study. Crit Care Med 2002; 30:368.

Pneumothorax

- **Essentials of Diagnosis**
  - Air in pleural space; described as percentage of chest cavity involved; open pneumothorax is associated with open sucking chest wound; tension pneumothorax causes shift in mediastinum toward contralateral lung
  - Spontaneous pneumothorax caused by pathologic process; rupture of bleb is most common
  - Male to female ratio is 6:1; age is commonly 16–24 years; patients at risk are tall, thin, smokers
  - Symptoms and signs include pleuritic chest pain, dyspnea, hypoxia, hypocapnia, diaphoresis, cyanosis, weakness, hypotension, cardiovascular collapse
  - Chest film is diagnostic
  - Pneumothorax of 1 cm on chest x-ray correlates with 25% loss of lung volume

- **Differential Diagnosis**
  - Ruptured bleb/chronic obstructive pulmonary disease
  - *Pneumocystis* pneumonia
  - Primary or metastatic lung tumor
  - Rupture of esophagus
  - Lung abscess
  - Cystic fibrosis

- **Treatment**
  - Small (<25%) and minimal symptoms: can be monitored conservatively
  - Larger asymptomatic, any symptomatic, increasing pneumothorax, or associated with effusion: insert chest tube
  - Indications for pleurodesis: air leaks >7 days, lung does not fully expand, high-risk occupation (scuba divers, pilots)
  - Complications: spontaneous recurrence in 50%, after 2 episodes in 75%, after 3 episodes in >80%

- **Pearl**

Reexpansion of lung is important because dead space in pleura can allow later infectious complications.

Reference

Etoch S et al: Tube thoracostomy. Arch Surg 1995;130:521.

Sarcoidosis

- **Essentials of Diagnosis**
  - Also known as Boeck sarcoid; benign lymphogranulomatous disease involving lungs, liver, spleen, lymph, skin, and bones; 20% have myocardial involvement, 30% have cutaneous involvement, 70% have hepatic and splenic involvement
  - Symptoms and signs may include nonspecific pulmonary symptoms (20–30%), including fever (15%) and cough; erythema nodosum may herald onset; others have weight loss, fatigue, weakness, malaise, enlarged lymph nodes (75%)
  - Chest film documents 5 stages: stage 0, no abnormality; stage 1, hilar or mediastinal adenopathy alone; stage 2, hilar adenopathy with pulmonary abnormalities; stage 3, diffuse pulmonary disease without adenopathy; stage 4, pulmonary fibrosis

- **Differential Diagnosis**
  - Hodgkin disease
  - Non-Hodgkin lymphoma

- **Treatment**
  - Asymptomatic patients: no therapy needed
  - Pulmonary impairment or symptoms: corticosteroids
  - Prognosis: long-term mortality may reach 10%

- **Pearl**

Sarcoidosis may be difficult to distinguish from malignant disease in the mediastinum.

Reference

Paramothayan S et al: Immunosuppressive and cytotoxic therapy for pulmonary sarcoidosis. Cochrane Database Syst Rev 2003;(3):CD003536.

Superior Vena Cava Syndrome

- **Essentials of Diagnosis**
  - 80–90% caused by malignant tumors: lung cancer (90%), thymoma, Hodgkin disease, lymphosarcoma, metastatic melanoma, breast or thyroid cancer; severity of symptoms correlates with pressure; azygous venous flow can increase to 35% of venous return (normal is 11%)
  - Symptoms and signs: nasal congestion is often the earliest symptom; swelling in face, arms, shoulders; blue or purple discoloration of skin; headache, nausea, dizziness, vomiting, vision changes, drowsiness, stupor
  - Venography determines location and extent of obstruction; aortography or CT scan excludes aortic aneurysm

- **Differential Diagnosis**
  - Angioneurotic edema
  - Congestive heart failure
  - Constrictive pericarditis

- **Treatment**
  - Cancer: diuretics, fluid restriction, head elevation, prompt radiation or chemotherapy; often subsides at 7–10 days of treatment
  - Benign tumors: surgical excision for incomplete obstruction
  - Radiotherapy is most effective for incomplete SVC obstruction
  - Prognosis: lung cancer with SVC obstruction has mean survival of 6–8 months; death rate from SVC obstruction is 1–2%

- **Pearl**

SVC syndrome is a poor prognostic sign for lung cancer.

Reference

Doty DB et al: Bypass of superior vena cava: Fifteen years' experience with spiral vein graft for obstruction of superior vena cava caused by benign disease. J Thorac Cardiovasc Surg 1990;99:889.

Thymic Carcinoma

- **Essentials of Diagnosis**
  - Rare variant of thymic lesions (<15%); biologically different from malignant thymoma; tends to be very invasive and aggressive; typically in young men (<50 years old)
  - Symptoms and signs: 50% of asymptomatic cases are identified on chest film; chest pain, dysphagia, dyspnea, or SVC syndrome most common if symptomatic
  - Chest film shows anterior mediastinal mass; CT scan is useful in assessing extent of lesion; magnetic resonance imaging can assess vascular invasion

- **Differential Diagnosis**
  - Rule out lymphoma; can be difficult to differentiate histologically from thymoma

- **Treatment**
  - Attempt complete resection
  - Medications: induction chemotherapy if not resectable; postoperative chemoradiation
  - Prognosis: high rate of recurrence locally and at distant sites; after thymectomy, 75% with myasthenia gravis are improved; 30% complete remission; younger patients (<40 years) do better after thymectomy

- **Pearl**

Evidence of local invasion (SVC syndrome, dysphagia, vocal cord paralysis) indicates a poor prognosis.

Reference

Rea F et al: Chemotherapy and operation for invasive thymoma. J Thorac Cardiovasc Surg 1993;106:543.

Thymoma & Myasthenia Gravis

- ■ Essentials of Diagnosis
  - Thymomas: most common type, often difficult to distinguish from lymphoma; 3 predominant cell types: lymphocytic (25%), epithelial (25%), lymphoepithelial (50%); 30% of patients with thymoma have myasthenia gravis
  - Myasthenia gravis: neuromuscular disorder of weakness and fatigability of voluntary muscles; decreased number of acetylcholine receptors at neuromuscular junctions; believed to be autoimmune process; thymoma develops in 15% of these patients
  - In myasthenia gravis, 90% of patients have serum antibodies against acetylcholine receptors; 70% have germinal center formation on thymic biopsy
  - CT scan is useful in assessing extent of lesion

- ■ Differential Diagnosis
  - Do not biopsy small, well-encapsulated mediastinal masses
  - Rule out lymphoma; can be difficult to differentiate histologically from thymoma
  - Thymic carcinoma: very aggressive variant of thymic lesions

- ■ Treatment
  - Thymoma: total thymectomy; cervical incision not useful for malignant disease, only benign disease
  - Aggressive resection is indicated for stages I, II, III; postoperative radiation therapy indicated for stage II
  - Myasthenia gravis: anticholinesterase drugs are initial treatment and used aggressively in postoperative period; corticosteroids used in selected cases; plasmapheresis can minimize need for anticholinesterase agents; early thymectomy may be indicated
  - Prognosis: myasthenia gravis has no bearing on prognosis; 10-year survival: stage I, 100%; stage II, 75%; stage III, 25%; stage IV, poor

- ■ Pearl

Complete thymectomy is necessary for malignant lesions.

Reference

Park HS et al: Thymoma. A retrospective study of 87 cases. Cancer 1994;73:2491.

Tietze Syndrome

- **Essentials of Diagnosis**
  - Painful, nonsuppurative inflammation of costochondral cartilage; unknown cause; may represent seronegative rheumatic disease
  - Symptoms and signs include local swelling, tenderness in parasternal area
  - Bone scan can localize inflamed costochondral junctions

- **Differential Diagnosis**
  - Rule out costochondral neoplasm if symptoms last >3 weeks
  - Other causes of breast pain

- **Treatment**
  - If symptoms are not self-limited, give nonsteroidal anti-inflammatory drugs, local or systemic corticosteroids
  - Surgery is indicated if symptoms last >3 weeks and mass is present, suggesting neoplasm

- **Pearl**

Tietze syndrome may be a persistent symptom complex despite attempts at therapy.

Reference

Aeschlimann A, Kahn MF: Tietze's syndrome: A critical review. Clin Exp Rheumatol 1990;8:407.

Tuberculosis, Pulmonary

- **Essentials of Diagnosis**
  - Gram-positive rods, often dormant but remain alive for the life of the host; initial infection affects mid zone of lungs, causing caseation in a few weeks; latent disease occurs when dormant tubercles reactivate in elderly or immunocompromised patients
  - 95% of cases are due to infection with *Mycobacterium tuberculosis, M bovis*, and *M avium-intracellulare*
  - Symptoms and signs: minimal symptoms in many patients or fever, cough; anorexia, weight loss; night sweats, excessive perspiration; chest pain; lethargy, fatigue
  - Chest film demonstrates involvement of apical and posterior upper lobes (85%)

- **Differential Diagnosis**
  - Bronchogenic carcinoma
  - Fungal infections such as histoplasmosis

- **Treatment**
  - Multidrug regimens including isoniazid, rifampin, pyrazinamide, ethambutol
  - Role of surgery has diminished dramatically
  - Surgery is indicated for failure of medical therapy, performance of diagnostic procedures, destroyed lung or cavitary lesions, postoperative complications, persistent bronchopleural fistula, intractable hemorrhage
  - Medications: isoniazid, streptomycin, ethambutol, rifampin
  - Prognosis: mortality is 10% with medical treatment; perioperative mortality is 1–10%; relapse rate is 4%

- **Pearl**

Drug-resistant TB has made therapy complicated in some regions.

Reference

Bass JB Jr et al: Treatment of tuberculosis and tuberculosis infection in adults and children. Am J Respir Crit Care Med 1994;149:1359.

10

Adult Cardiac Surgery

Aortic Stenosis

- **Essentials of Diagnosis**
  - Aortic valve is usually tricuspid; composed of fibrous skeleton, 3 cusps, and sinuses of Valsalva; during systole, eddy currents in sinuses of Valsalva prevent occlusion of coronary ostia; during diastole, cusps fall closed and coapt, supporting ejected column of blood
  - Aortic stenosis (AS) can be subvalvular, valvular, or supravalvular
  - Causes include congenital unicuspid or bicuspid valve, congenital subvalvular or supravalvular stenosis, rheumatic heart disease, degenerative fibrosis and calcification (most common)
  - Symptoms and signs: usually asymptomatic for years; triad of angina, syncope, congestive heart failure (CHF); CHF is late finding and ominous sign; harsh midsystolic murmur: second intercostal space along left sternal border, radiating to carotid arteries, not axilla or apex
  - Transesophageal echocardiography evaluates calcification, valve mobility, bicuspid anatomy, left ventricular (LV) hypertrophy, ejection fraction, valvular gradients, aortic regurgitation
  - Aortic valve area: mild AS, >1.5 cm^2; moderate AS, 1–1.5 cm^2; severe AS, ≤1 cm^2

- **Differential Diagnosis**
  - Causes of valve disease: rheumatic carditis (most common), valve collagen degeneration, infection
  - Less common causes: collagen-vascular disease, tumors, carcinoid syndrome, Marfan syndrome

- **Treatment**
  - Balloon valvotomy has limited role because high restenosis rate within 6 months; valve replacement is mechanical or porcine
  - Surgery is indicated for symptomatic AS with life expectancy of 1–3 years without intervention; asymptomatic with aortic valve gradient >50 mm Hg, or area ≤1 cm^2
  - Prognosis: operative mortality is <5%; 5-year survival is >85%; 50% of late deaths are noncardiac

- **Pearl**

Aortic stenosis triad: angina, syncope, and CHF.

Reference

Smedira NG et al: Balloon aortic valvuloplasty as a bridge to aortic valve replacement in critically ill patients. Ann Thorac Surg 1993;55:914.

Aortic Valve Regurgitation

- ■ Essentials of Diagnosis
  - • Aortic valve is usually tricuspid; composed of fibrous skeleton, 3 cusps, and sinuses of Valsalva; during systole, eddy currents in sinuses of Valsalva prevent occlusion of coronary ostia; during diastole, cusps fall closed and coapt, supporting ejected column of blood
  - • Aortic regurgitation (AR) is caused by abnormal coaptation of valve leaflets, allowing blood to return from aorta to ventricle during diastole
  - • Symptoms and signs: acute AR is poorly tolerated; causes severe pulmonary edema, CHF; if diastolic murmur is absent, indicates complete valve incompetence
  - • Chronic AR: early disease is asymptomatic; orthopnea, paroxysmal dyspnea, CHF develop later; wide pulse pressure, low diastolic pressure (Corrigan pulse); blowing high-pitched diastolic murmur heard at left lower sternal border at full expiration
  - • Echocardiography demonstrates LV function, chamber size, degree of regurgitation; catheterization defines degree of AR and coronary artery, aortic root anatomy

- ■ Differential Diagnosis
  - • Causes of chronic AR: rheumatic dilatation, annuloaortic ectasia, cystic medial necrosis, atherosclerosis, syphilis, arthritic inflammatory disease, congenital bicuspid valve
  - • Causes of acute AR: endocarditis, acute aortic dissection, trauma

- ■ Treatment
  - • Vasodilator therapy: useful in asymptomatic patients
  - • Selected patients can have valve repair with subcommissural annuloplasty if the lesion is simple annular dilatation
  - • Surgery to replace valve is indicated before onset of irreversible LV dilatation
  - • Prognosis: medical therapy for severe AR gives 5- and 10-year mortality of 25% and 50%, respectively; 5-year survival postoperatively with normal LV function is 85%; abnormal LV function decreases long-term survival

- ■ Pearl

Acute AR is poorly tolerated because of heart failure; ventricular dilatation in chronic AR is irreversible.

Reference

Dujardin KS et al: Mortality and morbidity of aortic regurgitation in clinical practice. A long-term follow-up study. Circulation 1999;99:1851.

Cardiac Tumors

- **Essentials of Diagnosis**
  - Myxoma: 75% of benign primary cardiac tumors; appearance ranges from smooth, round, firm encapsulated mass to loose conglomeration of gelatinous material; primary tumors of heart are rare: 0.002–0.3% of autopsies
  - Symptoms and signs vary depending on type and location of tumor; malignant tumors cause rapidly progressive CHF from valvular or myocardial infiltration; myxoma causes fever, weight loss, anemia, systemic embolization
  - Laboratory findings in myxoma include abnormal erythrocyte sedimentation rate, gamma globulin, liver aminotransferases
  - Transesophageal echocardiography is best choice for imaging; magnetic resonance imaging and computed tomography may be helpful for infiltrative lesions

- **Differential Diagnosis**
  - Myxoma
  - Metastatic tumors
  - Rare primary tumors

- **Treatment**
  - Most benign lesions are resectable and curable
  - Myxomas: cardiopulmonary bypass required; resect tumor and rim of normal tissue around attachment stalk
  - Resection for cardiac sarcomas and metastatic lesions is usually done for diagnosis; occasionally palliative
  - Prognosis: operative mortality is <1%; long-term survival for malignant cardiac lesions remains poor

- **Pearl**

Primary cardiac tumors are rare, but can include sarcoma, pheochromocytoma, and gastrinoma in addition to myxoma.

Reference

Shapiro LM: Cardiac tumors: Diagnosis and management. Heart 2001;85:218.

Cardiomyopathy, Idiopathic

- **Essentials of Diagnosis**
  - Unknown etiology; cause is often multifactorial; large, dilated heart with poor ventricular function
  - Symptoms and signs include those of heart failure
  - Workup: perform physical examination, electrocardiography, echocardiography

- **Differential Diagnosis**
  - Other causes of heart failure, including valvular heart disease

- **Treatment**
  - Cardiac transplantation may give best long-term results; mitral valve annuloplasty if enlarged annulus from LV enlargement; Batista procedure: ventricular reduction; limited use; biventricular pacing: restores normal depolarization to ventricles, increasing ejection fraction significantly
  - Prognosis: Batista procedure achieves limited survival, high mortality; medical therapy carries dismal prognosis

- **Pearl**

Cardiac transplantation may give the best long-term results for severe cardiomyopathy, but the small organ supply limits application.

Reference

Braile DM et al: Dynamic cardiomyoplasty: Long-term clinical results in patients with dilated cardiomyopathy. Ann Thorac Surg 2000;69:1445.

Cardiomyopathy, Ischemic

- ■ Essentials of Diagnosis
  - Coronary artery disease responsible for 20% of deaths; cardiovascular disease accounts for >40% of all deaths
  - Risk factors include smoking (secondhand smoke increases death rate from coronary disease by 30%; smoking cessation decreases coronary risk by 50% after 1 year of abstinence), hypercholesterolemia, male sex, diabetes mellitus, hypertension, family history
  - Symptoms and signs include retrosternal chest pain with pressure, choking, tightness; frequently radiates down left arm, left neck, occasionally right arm, mandible, ear; stable, progressive, or unstable angina; pulmonary edema from ischemia (poor prognosis)
  - Coronary angiography has highest sensitivity and specificity of any test (10% of disease underestimated)

- ■ Differential Diagnosis
  - Gastroesophageal reflux disease
  - Aneurysm
  - Aortic dissection

- ■ Treatment
  - Risk reduction: smoking cessation, hypertension control, lipid reduction
  - Percutaneous transluminal coronary angioplasty is >90% successful, but repeat interventions are common
  - Complete revascularization associated with improved outcome
  - Conventional CABG: internal mammary (preferred), saphenous vein, or radial artery used to bypass on average 3–4 coronary vessels
  - Minimally invasive: off-pump coronary artery bypass
  - Transmyocardial laser revascularization: for inoperable coronary disease; >70% symptomatic improvement; no change in survival
  - Surgery is indicated for severe or progressive angina despite medical therapy; refractory unstable angina
  - Medications: nitroglycerin, β-blockers, calcium channel blockers, aspirin
  - Prognosis: with CABG, 5- and 10-year survival is 92% and 81%, respectively

- ■ Pearl

Coronary artery disease accounts for at least 20% of all deaths.

Reference

Myers WO et al: CASS Registry long term surgical survival. Coronary Artery Surgery Study. J Am Coll Cardiol 1999;33:488.

Endocarditis

- **Essentials of Diagnosis**
  - Subacute: symptoms persist for months, usually caused by hemolytic streptococci
  - Acute or fulminant: symptoms for days to weeks, typically caused by *Staphylococcus aureus*
  - Symptoms and signs include fever, bacteremia, peripheral emboli; immunologic vascular phenomena: glomerulonephritis, Osler nodes (painful, erythematous nodules on pulp of fingers), Roth spots (retinal hemorrhages), subungual splinter hemorrhages, peripheral hemorrhages; Janeway lesions: flat, painless red spots on palms and soles of feet
  - Laboratory tests: 3 sets of blood cultures 1 hour apart are positive
  - Echocardiography documents location and degree of valve involvement, vegetation size, annular abscess

- **Differential Diagnosis**
  - Other sites of endovascular infection
  - Secondary effects on cardiac muscle function

- **Treatment**
  - Intravenous antibiotics
  - Surgery is indicated for severe valvular regurgitation with heart failure, abscess of valve annulus, persistent bacteremia >7 days despite adequate antibiotic therapy, fungal or gram-negative bacterial infection, recurrent emboli, mobile vegetations >1 cm
  - Prognosis: if untreated, mortality is nearly 100%; with parenteral antibiotics, mortality is 30–50%; with antibiotics and surgery, overall mortality is 10%

- **Pearl**

Classic physical examination findings include Osler nodes, Janeway lesions, and Roth spots.

Reference

Bayer AS et al: Diagnosis and management of infective endocarditis and its complications. Circulation 1998;98:2936.

Mitral Regurgitation

- ■ Essentials of Diagnosis
  - • Causes include rheumatic heart disease, idiopathic mitral valve (MV) calcification, mitral valve prolapse, infective endocarditis, ischemic mitral regurgitation (MR), postinfarction papillary muscle rupture (0.1% of coronary artery disease)
  - • Symptoms and signs include exertional dyspnea, orthopnea, fatigue; symptoms do not correlate with degree of MR; hemoptysis; atrial fibrillation (75% of severe cases); malaise, fever, chills may indicate infective endocarditis, CHF with new murmur days after myocardial infarction (MI), high-pitched holosystolic murmur radiating to axilla and back
  - • Transesophageal echocardiography locates regurgitation jet; cardiac catheterization demonstrates left atrial v waves, elevated LV pressure; cardiac index <2.0 L/min/m^2 and wide arteriovenous oxygen difference indicate severe impairment

- ■ Differential Diagnosis
  - • Endocarditis
  - • Secondary LV dysfunction

- ■ Treatment
  - • Preload reduction with diuretics, afterload reduction with angiotensin-converting enzyme (ACE) inhibitors
  - • Virtually all mitral valve prolapses can be repaired with posterior leaflet reconstruction and annuloplasty
  - • Surgery is indicated for symptomatic heart failure (New York Heart Association class II or greater); or if asymptomatic, ejection fraction $<60\%$, end-systolic dimension >45 mm, pulmonary hypertension, or new atrial fibrillation
  - • Medications: diuretics, ACE inhibitors reduce afterload and MR
  - • Prognosis: operative mortality, 2–5%; 5- and 10-year survival, 80% and 65%, respectively; survival better for MV repair than for replacement

- ■ Pearl

Acute papillary muscle rupture can create mitral regurgitation, complicating an acute myocardial infarction.

Reference

Enriquez-Sarano M et al: Valve repair improves the outcome of surgery for mitral regurgitation. A multivariate analysis. Circulation 1995;91:1022.

Mitral Stenosis

- ■ Essentials of Diagnosis
  - Mitral stenosis (MS): fibrosis and narrowing of valvular area causing ventricular inflow obstruction during diastole
  - Symptoms and signs include dyspnea (initially with exertion), orthopnea; atrial fibrillation with atrial dilation, often with clinical deterioration from dependence on atrial kick (20% of cardiac output) and tachycardia; thin cachetic "mitral facies"; peripheral edema, hepatic enlargement, hepatojugular reflux; opening snap of MV from tensing of leaflets by chordae (heard best at apex); diastolic low-pitched rumbling murmur (heard best at apex), accentuated if in sinus rhythm with atrial contraction
  - Echocardiography and catheterization give information on valve anatomy and area; normal mitral area = 3 cm^2/m^2 body surface area; significant MS is ≤1 cm^2/m^2 body surface area

- ■ Differential Diagnosis
  - Causes of valve disease: rheumatic carditis (most common), valve collagen degeneration, infection
  - Less common causes: collagen-vascular disease, tumors, carcinoid syndrome, Marfan syndrome

- ■ Treatment
  - Asymptomatic MS: treat medically with heart rate control, anticoagulation for atrial fibrillation
  - Moderate to severe symptomatic MS: percutaneous balloon valvotomy; ideal for minimally calcified valve with no MR; surgical commissurotomy (50%) if no calcification
  - Surgery is indicated for all symptomatic patients, significant pulmonary hypertension, pulmonary edema, new-onset atrial fibrillation, episodes of thromboembolism
  - Prognosis: 10-year survival in asymptomatic patients >80%; survival for symptomatic patients 15%; percutaneous balloon valvotomy: stenosis-free survival at 10 years, 56%; operative mortality for isolated MV procedures, 1–5%; repeat operations necessary in 2–4% per year

- ■ Pearl
  Signs include dyspnea, orthopnea, and tachycardia.

Reference

Bonow RO et al: Guidelines for the management of patients with valvular heart disease: Executive summary. A report of the American College of Cardiology/American Heart Association Task Force on Practice Guidelines (Committee on Management of Patients with Valvular Heart Disease). Circulation 1998;98:1949.

Tricuspid Valve Disease

■ Essentials of Diagnosis

- Functional tricuspid disease: secondary to right ventricular (RV) dilation causing enlargement of free-wall tricuspid annulus; reflects and further worsens RV failure; carcinoid involvement of tricuspid valve causes fibrotic deposits on leaflets
- Symptoms and signs: tricuspid stenosis (TS) and tricuspid regurgitation (TR) related to degree of systemic venous hypertension; fatigue, weakness, no signs of pulmonary congestion; TS: prominent A wave if in sinus rhythm; TR: accentuated jugular V wave; TR with MV disease: pulmonary hypertension, RV failure, rapid deterioration
- Echocardiography shows anatomy and severity of regurgitation, RV function, and cause; cardiac catheterization diagnoses disease and identifies cause

■ Differential Diagnosis

- Causes of valve disease: rheumatic carditis (most common), valve collagen degeneration, infection
- Less common causes: collagen-vascular disease, tumors, carcinoid syndrome, Marfan syndrome

■ Treatment

- Rheumatic TS: commissurotomy or valve replacement (residual gradients tolerated poorly)
- Symptomatic carcinoid: replace valve
- Tricuspid endocarditis: many patients have septic pulmonary emboli; give antibiotics; replace valve with allograft
- Surgery is indicated for MV disease requiring operation; symptomatic disease

■ Pearl

Carcinoid heart disease is often progressive and may require valve replacement.

Reference

Bonow RO et al: Guidelines for the management of patients with valvular heart disease: Executive summary. A report of the American College of Cardiology/American Heart Association Task Force on Practice Guidelines (Committee on Management of Patients with Valvular Heart Disease). Circulation 1998;98:1949.

Ventricular Septal Defect (VSD)

- ■ Essentials of Diagnosis
    - Postinfarct VSD: infarction of interventricular septum with subsequent VSD formation; interval between MI and septal rupture is 1–12 days; classically, sudden shock or congestive heart failure develops in a patient after MI; VSD occurs in <1% of patients with acute MI
    - LV aneurysm: large MI progresses to thinned-out transmural scar, bulges paradoxically during systole; 90% of aneurysms involve anteroseptal LV and 10% posterior; occurs after 2–4% of MIs; incidence is decreasing with more aggressive management of MI
    - Symptoms and signs: postinfarct VSD causes harsh holosystolic murmur along left sternal border; 67% have palpable thrill; LV aneurysm causes congestive heart failure, angina, embolization, ventricular dysrhythmias, prominent apical pulse
    - Echocardiography and catheterization are definitive for postinfarct VSD and LV aneurysm

- ■ Differential Diagnosis
    - Papillary muscle dysfunction; rupture of papillary muscle with acute mitral insufficiency
    - Pericardial friction rub after MI (Dressler syndrome)

- ■ Treatment
    - Postinfarct VSD: preoperative intra-aortic balloon pump; surgical patch closure of VSD (using double patch) plus coronary artery bypass performed early
    - LV aneurysm: resect aneurysm (Dor procedure) plus coronary revascularization
    - Surgery is indicated for postinfarct VSD in nearly all cases; for LV aneurysm when good to moderate operative risk
    - Prognosis: postinfarct VSD has poor prognosis; 24% die on first day, 65% by 2 weeks, 81% by 2 months; 50–80% survive operation depending on degree of multiorgan failure; for LV aneurysm, survival is dictated by underlying myocardial function

- ■ Pearl

The best treatment is prevention by limiting the scope of myocardial damage from MI.

Reference

Chaux AC et al: Postinfarction ventricular septal defect. Semin Thorac Cardiovasc Surg 1998;10:93.

11

Congenital Cardiac Surgery

Aortic Coarctation & Interrupted Aortic Arch, Congenital

- **Essentials of Diagnosis**
  - Aortic coarctation: 98% located near aortic isthmus (proximal to ductus arteriosus); associated anomalies occur in 70% of neonates, 15% of older children: patent foramen ovale, patent ductus arteriosus (PDA), ventricular septal defect (VSD), bicuspid aortic valve (40%), Shone syndrome
  - Interrupted aortic arch: type A (35%), absence of arch distal to left subclavian artery; type B (60%), between left carotid and left subclavian artery; type C (5%), between innominate and left carotid artery
  - Symptoms and signs: aortic coarctation causes 2 distinct presentations: in early infancy, severe congestive heart failure, sudden cardiovascular collapse with duct closure; in older children, many are asymptomatic or have headache, leg claudication with running, frequent nosebleeds, hypertension of upper extremities, left ventricular (LV) hypertrophy
  - Interrupted aortic arch: symptomatic in first few days of life
  - Chest film for aortic coarctation shows reversed "3" sign; echocardiography and magnetic resonance imaging are diagnostic

- **Differential Diagnosis**
  - Evaluate for other cardiac or extracardiac anomalies

- **Treatment**
  - Aortic coarctation: in neonates, alprostadil (prostaglandin E_1 [PGE_1]) to maintain ductus patency, mechanical ventilation, HCO_3
  - Resect with end-to-end anastomosis, subclavian flap aortoplasty with or without resection, patch aortoplasty, interposition graft, percutaneous balloon
  - Interrupted aortic arch: PGE_1 maintains hemodynamics; surgery is indicated as soon as patient is stabilized
  - Prognosis for aortic coarctation: if untreated, mortality is 50% by age 30 years; 5-year survival 95% but can be low (40%) if intracardiac anomaly; postoperative hypertension usually resolves in several days but should be treated aggressively

- **Pearl**

Always evaluate for other cardiac abnormalities.

Reference

Conte S et al: Surgical management of neonatal coarctation. J Thorac Cardiovasc Surg 1995;109:663.

Atrial Septal Defect

- **Essentials of Diagnosis**
  - Ostium secundum type: most common and largest atrial septal defect (ASD)
  - "Sinus venosus defect": located high in atrial septum, associated with partial anomalous pulmonary venous return
  - Eisenmenger syndrome: increased pulmonary hypertension to such extent that left-to-right shunt ceases and shunt becomes right to left, requiring heart-lung transplantation
  - Symptoms and signs: acyanotic, often asymptomatic; S2 widely split and fixed; pulmonary systolic ejection murmur; diastolic flow murmur at left lower sternal border
  - Echocardiography is diagnostic

- **Differential Diagnosis**
  - Evaluate for other cardiac or extracardiac anomalies

- **Treatment**
  - Most ASDs should be closed; optimal time is debated; many are now closed percutaneously (patient must weigh ≥10 kg)
  - Surgery is indicated for presence of ASD in low- to moderate-risk patient
  - Prognosis is excellent

- **Pearl**

Always evaluate for other cardiac anomalies.

Reference

Berger F et al: Comparison of results and complications of surgical and Amplatzer device closure of atrial septal defects. J Thorac Cardiovasc Surg 1999;118:674.

Atrioventricular Canal Defect

■ Essentials of Diagnosis
- Range of defects is possible
- Partial atrioventricular (AV) canal defect: septum primum ASD, deficient lower atrial septum only
- Transitional AV canal defect: intermediate form with ASD and minor deficiency in upper ventricular system
- Complete AV canal defect: ASD and severe valve anomalies
- Eisenmenger syndrome: increased pulmonary hypertension to such extent that left-to-right shunt ceases and shunt becomes right to left, requiring heart-lung transplantation
- Symptoms and signs include heart failure in infancy, cardiomegaly, blowing pansystolic murmur (varies), loud S_2, fixed split
- Echocardiography is best for diagnosis

■ Differential Diagnosis
- Must define the extent of canal defect to plan correction

■ Treatment
- Inhaled nitric oxide, oxygen, or intravenous tolazoline reverses pulmonary artery (PA) vasoconstriction
- Timing of correction indicated by degree of anomaly and symptoms; partial defect takes patch closure; complete defect requires patch closure of septal defects and reconstruction of valves
- Surgery is indicated by 6 months of age for complete defect; by 1 year of age for less severe types
- Prognosis: mortality varies with defect and age; for partial defect, 10-year survival is 98%; for complete defect, operative mortality is 3–5%; 10-year survival is 90%

■ Pearl

Always evaluate for other congenital abnormalities.

Reference

Anderson RH et al: The diagnostic features of atrioventricular septal defect with common atrioventricular junction. Cardiol Young 1998;8:33.

Double-Outlet Right Ventricle

- ■ Essentials of Diagnosis
  - Double-outlet right ventricle: both great arteries (50% of annulus of each valve) arise from right ventricle; uncommon and extremely complex; location of VSD (always present) determines classification
  - Single ventricle: 1 ventricular chamber receiving blood from both tricuspid and mitral valves; associated with abnormal great vessel arrangements, 85%; common AV valve, 30%; stenosis or regurgitation of AV valve, 25%; pulmonary stenosis or atresia, 50%; aortic stenosis, 33%; situs inversus, dextrocardia, and asplenia, 20%
  - Symptoms and signs: in double-outlet right ventricle, symptoms depend on location of VSD and degree of outflow obstruction; in single ventricle, symptoms vary based on amount of pulmonary and systemic blood flow
  - Workup: perform echocardiography, catheterization

- ■ Differential Diagnosis
  - Thoroughly evaluate for other congenital defects

- ■ Treatment
  - Double-outlet right ventricle: create intraventricular baffle to direct LV flow to aorta, closing septal defect and avoiding subpulmonary obstruction
  - Single ventricle: initially, shunt or PA band, ventricular partitioning, then staged correction toward Fontan procedure
  - Prognosis: double-outlet right ventricle: 10-year survival, 60–80%; single ventricle: 1-year survival, 40–80%

- ■ Pearl
  Always evaluate for other congenital abnormalities.

Reference
Takeuchi K et al: Surgical outcome of double-outlet right ventricle with sub-pulmonary VSD. Ann Thorac Surg 2001;71:49.

Heart Lesions, Congenital

■ **Essentials of Diagnosis**
- Anomalous left coronary artery (LCA): LCA arises from PA
- Pulmonary arteriovenous fistula: rare anomaly, associated with Rendu-Osler-Weber syndrome in 50%
- Persistent left superior vena cava (LSVC): LSVC connects left jugular and subclavian veins to coronary sinus; relatively common anomaly
- Endocardial fibroelastosis: inoperable lesion; associated with aortic coarctation, aortic stenosis, anomalous LCA, mitral valve disease
- Cardiac tumors: uncommon in children; primary tumors more common than metastatic lesions; >90% are benign
- Symptoms and signs: LCA causes pallor, sweating, tachycardia, episodic chest pain suggesting angina pectoris; pulmonary arteriovenous fistula causes dyspnea, cyanosis, right heart failure occasionally in infants; cyanosis, clubbing, polycythemia in late childhood; LSVC is usually asymptomatic; endocardial fibroelastosis causes left heart failure; cardiac tumors produce symptoms from space-occupying lesion or involvement of conduction system

■ **Differential Diagnosis**
- Other congenital heart lesions

■ **Treatment**
- LCA: anastomosis of LCA to aorta
- Pulmonary arteriovenous fistula: fistula excision and local pulmonary resection or formal lobectomy
- LSVC: if adequate drainage to right side, ligate LSVC
- Endocardial fibroelastosis: cardiac transplantation is the only option
- Cardiac tumors: transvenous biopsy for asymptomatic or limited symptoms, then attempt complete removal of tumor, preserving critical structures
- Rhabdomyoma: spontaneous regression considered normal

■ **Pearl**
Always evaluate for other congenital cardiac defects.

Reference

Laks H et al: Aortic implantation of anomalous left coronary artery: An improved surgical approach. J Thorac Cardiovasc Surg 1995;109:519.

Heart Lesions, Congenital: Increased Pulmonary Flow

- **Essentials of Diagnosis**
  - Congenital heart lesion that increases PA blood flow results in left-to-right shunt, lung infection, pulmonary vascular congestion, PA hypertension, right heart failure
  - Aortopulmonary window: findings similar to PDA; early heart failure and pulmonary hypertension
  - Ruptured sinus of Valsalva: continuous, well-localized parasternal murmur with associated thrill; rapid heart failure develops in most patients
  - LV-right atrial shunt: heart failure in infancy or late childhood; murmur is not diagnostic
  - Coronary artery fistula: many asymptomatic, or myocardial ischemia or heart failure, continuous murmur over heart

- **Differential Diagnosis**
  - Evaluate for other congenital cardiac anomalies

- **Treatment**
  - Aortopulmonary window: surgical repair with patch closure
  - Ruptured sinus of Valsalva: early operation warranted
  - LV-right atrial shunt: closed primarily on bypass
  - Coronary artery fistula: ligate fistulous connections without interrupting coronary artery
  - Prognosis: low operative mortality rate for LV-right atrial shunt and coronary artery fistula

- **Pearl**

Always evaluate for associated congenital anomalies.

Reference

Rabinovitch M: Pathobiology of pulmonary hypertension: Impact on clinical management. Semin Thorac Cardiovasc Surg Pediatr Card Surg Annu 2000;3:63.

Hypoplastic Left Heart Syndrome

- **Essentials of Diagnosis**
  - Obstructive congenital heart lesion; spectrum of underdevelopment of left-sided structures (mitral and aortic valves, left ventricle, ascending aorta, and arch); commonly associated with mitral and aortic valve atresia, LV hypoplasia; ascending aorta measures 2–3.5 cm
  - Symptoms and signs: with closure of ductus, causes respiratory failure, hemodynamic failure, acidosis, multisystem organ failure
  - Echocardiography is sufficient for diagnosis

- **Differential Diagnosis**
  - Evaluate for other cardiac and extracardiac anomalies

- **Treatment**
  - Initial management: mechanical ventilation, fluids, pressor and HCO_3 resuscitation; maintain ductal patency with PGE_1; if inadequate mixing, perform balloon atrial septostomy
  - Staged surgical procedure: Norwood, followed by Glenn or hemi-Fontan at 6–8 months, followed by Fontan at 1–1.5 years
  - Cardiac transplantation
  - Prognosis: improved recently; 5-year survival, 40–70%; most deaths occur soon after first stage

- **Pearl**

Evaluate for other congenital anomalies.

Reference

Weldner PW et al: The Norwood operation and subsequent Fontan operation in infants with complex congenital heart disease. J Thorac Cardiovasc Surg 1995;109:654.

Mitral Valve Disease, Congenital

- **Essentials of Diagnosis**
  - Congenital mitral valve disease: uncommon; can result in stenosis or insufficiency; wide spectrum of disease; most patients have associated anomalies
  - Stenosis: supravalvular ring, parachute mitral valve, subaortic stenosis, aortic coarctation
  - Insufficiency: dilated annulus, shortened chordae, restricted leaflets
  - Cor triatriatum: rare anomaly; pulmonary veins enter accessory venous chamber demarcated from true left atrium by a diaphragm; LSVC common; results in pulmonary venous hypertension, pulmonary congestion, elevated PA pressures

- **Differential Diagnosis**
  - Evaluate for other cardiac or extracardiac anomalies

- **Treatment**
  - Congenital mitral valve disease: valve repair preferred over valve replacement if possible; ensure adequate heart function before leaving operating room
  - Cor triatriatum: surgical excision of membrane corrects abnormality
  - Prognosis: good for cor triatriatum

- **Pearl**

Always evaluate for associated congenital anomalies.

Reference

Yoshimura N et al: Surgery for mitral valve disease in the pediatric age group. J Thorac Cardiovasc Surg 1999;118:99.

Patent Ductus Arteriosus

■ Essentials of Diagnosis

- Results in left-to-right shunt, pulmonary vascular congestion, PA hypertension, lung infection, right heart failure, pulmonary vaso-constriction, pulmonary vascular obstructive disease
- Associated with other anomalies; 5% of patients with untreated PDA die of heart and pulmonary failure by age 1 year
- Symptoms and signs: infants have poor feeding, respiratory distress, frequent respiratory infection, heart failure; older patients are often asymptomatic or have continuous murmur over pulmonary area, loud S_2, bounding peripheral pulses

■ Differential Diagnosis

- Primary pulmonary dysfunction from prematurity

■ Treatment

- Premature infants: medical therapy with indomethacin (50% success)
- Term infants or children: surgical obliteration by ligation, clipping, or division
- Larger infants and children: video thoracoscopy
- PA band is palliative and can reduce PA flow to alleviate RV failure and progression of pulmonary hypertension
- Medications: indomethacin (PG inhibitor) 50% successful; efficacy decreases with age
- Prognosis: operative mortality is near 0%; recurrence rate is <1% among patients treated surgically

■ Pearl

Always evaluate for associated congenital anomalies.

Reference

Hawkins JA et al: Cost and efficacy of surgical ligation versus transcatheter coil occlusion of patent ductus arteriosus. J Thorac Cardiovasc Surg 1996; 112:1634.

Pulmonary Atresia

- **Essentials of Diagnosis**
  - Congenital heart lesion that decreases PA blood flow, resulting in right-to-left shunt; cyanosis and decreased oxygen delivery cause compensatory polycythemia (hematocrit >70%) and spontaneous thrombosis
  - Symptoms and signs include cyanosis at birth; duct closure causes profound hypoxia, acidosis
  - Chest film shows diminished flow into lungs; echocardiography is diagnostic; catheterization defines coronary anatomy, RV coronary circulation

- **Differential Diagnosis**
  - Echocardiography and catheterization are needed

- **Treatment**
  - ASD creation or ductus maintenance (with alprostadil) necessary for early survival
  - Surgical options to increase pulmonary flow: Blalock-Taussig shunt: subclavian artery to ipsilateral PA in end-to-side fashion; modified Blalock-Taussig shunt: subclavian to PA using polytetrafluoroethylene (PTFE); Glenn shunt: SVC to PA; Fontan: SVC and inferior vena cava (IVC) rerouted to PA
  - Prognosis: 1-year mortality, 10–20%; prognosis is improving

- **Pearl**

Always evaluate for associated congenital anomalies.

Reference

Jahangiri M et al: Improved results with selective management in pulmonary atresia with intact ventricular septum. J Thorac Cardiovasc Surg 1999;118:1046.

Pulmonary Stenosis, Congenital

- **Essentials of Diagnosis**
  - Pulmonary stenosis impedes forward blood flow and increases ventricular afterload; without VSD, obstructive lesion causes hypertrophy of corresponding ventricle; most patients have patent foramen ovale
  - Symptoms and signs include poor feeding, hypoxic spells, occasionally sudden death; older children may be asymptomatic or have fatigue, dyspnea on exertion, dizziness, angina; murmur easily detected

- **Differential Diagnosis**
  - Evaluate for other cardiac or extracardiac anomalies

- **Treatment**
  - Neonates: PGE_1 (alprostadil) maintains PDA until pulmonary valve obstruction is relieved
  - Surgery: for isolated pulmonary stenosis, catheter balloon dilation is >90% successful; if catheter intervention unsuccessful, perform surgical valvotomy (may need transannular patch or systemic to pulmonary shunt)
  - Prognosis: >90% respond well to catheter or surgical therapy; for critical pulmonary stenosis, mortality is 3–10% after treatment; restenosis rate is 10–25%

- **Pearl**

Always evaluate for associated congenital anomalies.

Reference

Hanley FL et al: Outcomes in critically ill neonates with pulmonary stenosis and intact ventricular septum: A multiinstitutional study. Congenital Heart Surgeons Society. J Am Coll Cardiol 1993;22:183.

Pulmonary Venous Connection, Total Anomalous

- **Essentials of Diagnosis**
  - Three types (depending on site of connection): type I (supracardiac), left-sided vertical vein drains into innominate vein (45%); type II (cardiac), connection to right atrium or coronary sinus (25%); type III (infracardiac), connection to infradiaphragmatic IVC or portal vein (25%); 5% have mixed venous drainage
  - Pulmonary venous obstruction occurs in nearly all patients with infracardiac connection, <25% with supracardiac connection; obstruction leads to increased pulmonary vascular resistance; degree of obstruction determines clinical presentation

- **Differential Diagnosis**
  - Must distinguish type (I, II, III) to plan repair
  - Presence of other cardiac anomalies uncommon, but high mortality

- **Treatment**
  - Surgical repair in all cases; no effective medical therapy
  - Supracardiac and infracardiac: anastomosis of pulmonary venous confluence to left atrium, ligation of anomalous connection
  - Prognosis: mortality limited to patients with severe obstruction (10–15%) from pulmonary hypertension; patients with associated anomalies have high mortality (>30%); recurrence of pulmonary obstruction in 5–10%

- **Pearl**

Always evaluate for associated congenital anomalies.

Reference

Calderone CA et al: Surgical management of total anomalous pulmonary venous drainage: Impact of coexisting cardiac anomalies. Ann Thorac Surg 1998;66:1521.

Tetralogy of Fallot

- ■ Essentials of Diagnosis
  - • Four anomalies: VSD, pulmonary stenosis or atresia, overriding aorta, RV hypertrophy
  - • Pulmonary stenosis may involve infundibulum, valve, or main PA; pulmonary atresia or stenosis has wide spectrum of severity; pulmonary flow depends on aortopulmonary collaterals, can be extensive enough to cause congestive heart failure
  - • Symptoms and signs are related to amount of pulmonary blood flow; with closure of ductus, cyanosis and acidosis may be severe
  - • Echocardiography confirms diagnosis; catheterization is necessary to define size of PAs and identify aortopulmonary arteries

- ■ Differential Diagnosis
  - • Evaluate for other cardiac or extracardiac anomalies

- ■ Treatment
  - • Medications: alprostadil, HCO_3, oxygen
  - • One-stage surgical correction: patch repair of VSD, patch to infundibulum to widen outflow tract; pulmonary insufficiency tolerated in children, may be temporary
  - • Two-stage surgical correction: initial systemic-PA shunt, later definitive correction
  - • Tetralogy of Fallot with pulmonary atresia: connect large aortopulmonary shunts to RV outflow or to shunt; induces growth of vasculature
  - • Prognosis: RV dysfunction is common; mortality <5% with pulmonary stenosis, 30–45% with atresia; repeat operation on outflow tract, 10–15% at 10 years; of patients reaching adulthood, >90% employed, >50% exercise, >20% need cardiac medications

- ■ Pearl

Always evaluate for associated congenital anomalies.

Reference

Fraser CD et al: Tetralogy of Fallot: Surgical management individualized to the patient. Ann Thorac Surg 2001;71:1556.

Transposition of the Great Arteries

- **Essentials of Diagnosis**
  - Transposition of great arteries: aorta connected to morphologic right ventricle is most common (D-transposition); ASD and PDA common; VSD in 25%, more common in unusual arrangements
  - Corrected transposition of great arteries: L-transposition; right-sided morphologic left ventricle connected to PA, left-sided morphologic right ventricle connected to aorta; blood flow in series through right and left side, so oxygenated blood reaches systemic circulation; VSD in >75%, subpulmonary obstruction in 50%
  - Symptoms and signs: transposition causes cyanosis at birth, deterioration with duct closure, worsening hypoxia and acidosis; corrected transposition is uncommon in infancy; congestive heart failure eventually develops from pulmonary stenosis, tricuspid insufficiency
  - Echocardiography is diagnostic

- **Differential Diagnosis**
  - Evaluate for other cardiac or extracardiac anomalies

- **Treatment**
  - Mustard and Senning procedures: intra-atrial channels direct systemic venous return to left ventricle, pulmonary return to right ventricle
  - Arterial switch procedure: done with hypothermic cardiopulmonary bypass or hypothermic circulatory arrest; switches aorta and PA onto correct ventricles; coronary arteries also switched with aorta
  - Prognosis: if transposition untreated, 50% die within 1 month, 90% within 1 year; switch procedure gives <2% mortality; patients infrequently require further intervention; for corrected transposition, 10-year survival 50%

- **Pearl**

Always evaluate for associated congenital anomalies.

Reference

Alva C et al: The feasibility of complete anatomical correction in the setting of discordant atrioventricular connections. Br Heart J 1999;81:539.

Tricuspid Atresia

■ **Essentials of Diagnosis**

- Congenital heart lesion that decreases PA blood flow, resulting in right-to-left shunt; squatting increases systemic resistance, causing increased pulmonary flow and oxygen saturation
- Ebstein anomaly: septal and posterior leaflets of tricuspid valve small and displaced toward RV apex; portion of right ventricle thin and atrialized; associated ASD and patent foramen ovale
- Symptoms and signs: tricuspid atresia symptoms are related to degree of ASD/VSD restriction, great vessel anatomy; majority have some degree of cyanosis; no obstruction to systemic output; in Ebstein anomaly, cyanosis and arrhythmias common; 50% develop right heart failure, hypoxia, hepatomegaly, dysrhythmias
- Echocardiography is diagnostic; catheterization determines suitability for repair and potential correction of ASD

■ **Differential Diagnosis**

- Evaluate for other cardiac or extracardiac anomalies

■ **Treatment**

- Tricuspid atresia: ASD balloon septoplasty if restrictive; Blalock-Taussig shunt often done initially to provide pulmonary flow; Glenn shunt followed by Fontan procedure to complete 3-stage repair
- Ebstein anomaly: oversew atrialized portion of right ventricle, correct tricuspid valve incompetence (successful in 50% of cases); newer techniques involve correction of right ventricle and tricuspid valve
- Surgical options to increase pulmonary flow: Blalock-Taussig shunt: subclavian artery to ipsilateral PA in end-to-side fashion; modified Blalock-Taussig shunt: subclavian to PA using PTFE; Glenn: SVC to PA shunt; Fontan: SVC and IVC rerouted to PA

■ **Pearl**

Always evaluate for associated congenital anomalies.

Reference

Dearani JA et al: Congenital Heart Surgery Nomenclature and Database Project: Ebstein's anomaly and tricuspid valve disease. Ann Thorac Surg 2000;69:S106.

Truncus Arteriosus

- **Essentials of Diagnosis**
  - Single large truncal vessel overrides ventricular septum and distributes all blood ejected from heart; truncal root bifurcates into pulmonary trunk and aorta; VSD usually directly beneath truncal valve; ASD in >40%, interrupted aortic arch in 10%, abnormal origins of coronary artery; pulmonary flow usually increased
  - Symptoms and signs include heart failure in most, pulmonary vascular disease early

- **Differential Diagnosis**
  - Evaluate for associated cardiac and extracardiac anomalies

- **Treatment**
  - Surgical repair: close VSD, separate PAs from truncal root, place pulmonary allograft valve from right ventricle, correct truncal insufficiency
  - Surgery is indicated once diagnosis is made
  - Prognosis: operative mortality 5–30% (related to truncal valve insufficiency, interrupted arch, coronary anomalies, pulmonary hypertension); survivors often need future repair or replacement of truncal or pulmonary valve

- **Pearl**

Always evaluate for associated congenital anomalies.

Reference

Jahangiri M et al: Repair of the truncal valve and associated interrupted arch in neonates with truncus arteriosus. J Thorac Cardiovasc Surg 2000;119:508.

Ventricular Septal Defect, Congenital

- **Essentials of Diagnosis**
  - Defects occur in 4 anatomic positions: perimembranous septum (85%), anterior to crista supraventricularis, beneath leaflet of tricuspid valve, or in muscular septum
  - Often associated with more complex defects: truncus arteriosus, AV canal defect, tetralogy of Fallot, transposition of great arteries
  - Isolated perimembranous defects may have associated PDA, aortic coarctation; supracristal defects may have aortic regurgitation
  - Symptoms and signs: if defect is small, no symptoms; if large, defect causes heart failure with dyspnea, frequent respiratory infections, poor growth
  - Echocardiography is diagnostic

- **Differential Diagnosis**
  - May be part of a more complex defect (truncus arteriosus), AV canal defect, tetralogy of Fallot

- **Treatment**
  - 33% have small defects, which often close spontaneously by age 8 years; 33% have large defects (symptomatic), which require earlier treatment; asymptomatic defects unlikely to close spontaneously are closed when safe (larger infant or child; no other intervening medical conditions)
  - Surgery is indicated for medically refractory symptoms in infants, elevated PA pressure, canal-type defect or malaligned conoventricular defect, aortic insufficiency (supracristal defect)
  - Prognosis: operative mortality is rare; for severe preoperative failure, mortality is 3–5%; symptomatic improvement is dramatic; no change in pulmonary resistance

- **Pearl**

Always evaluate for associated congenital anomalies.

Reference

Jacobs JP et al: Congenital Heart Surgery Nomenclature and Database Project: Ventricular septal defect. Ann Thorac Surg 2000;69:S25.

12

Arteries

Abdominal Aortic Aneurysm

- **Essentials of Diagnosis**
  - Permanent aortic dilation ($\geq$50% increase in diameter); classified by etiology (degenerative, inflammatory, mechanical, congenital, dissecting) and by shape (saccular, fusiform); for abdominal aortic aneurysm (AAA) measuring 5.0–5.5 cm, rupture risk 40% at 5 years; usually ruptures posterolaterally to left
  - Infected (mycotic): bacterial contamination of preexisting aneurysm or weakness of infected aortic wall
  - Symptoms and signs: rarely produces symptoms if intact; painless, pulsatile abdominal mass above umbilicus; may be uncomfortable on palpation; severe pain caused by inflammatory or ruptured AAA or acute expansion; rupture causes sudden, severe abdominal or back pain radiating to back or inguinal area, faintness or syncope, shock
  - Triad for rupture: pain, pulsatile abdominal mass, hypotension (found in <67% of patients)
  - Ultrasound is inexpensive screening test, measures size and position; computed tomography (CT) scan is diagnostic, allows accurate sizing, provides information about surrounding anatomy

- **Differential Diagnosis**
  - Other causes upper abdominal masses: pancreas, kidney, liver
  - Other causes of hypotension

- **Treatment**
  - Open repair options: tube graft, bifurcated graft
  - Endovascular repair: evolving anatomic criteria; performed through open cutdown of femoral arteries
  - Surgery is indicated for AAA size >5–5.5 cm, depending on individual patient's risk
  - For small AAA not large enough to warrant repair, monitor with serial ultrasound every 6–12 months
  - Prognosis: operative mortality from ruptured AAA >60%, overall mortality is 90% as many patients die without operation

- **Pearl**

Endovascular management of AAA is evolving, as optimal strategies and anatomic requirements for preventing and treating AAA rupture with endovascular devices are assessed.

Reference

Moore WS et al: Abdominal aortic aneurysm: A 6-year comparison of endovascular versus transabdominal repair. Ann Surg 1999;230:298.

Aneurysms, Peripheral

- **Essentials of Diagnosis**
  - True aneurysm: involves all 3 layers of vessel wall
  - False aneurysm (pseudoaneurysm): disruption of artery causing contained hematoma confined by fibrous capsule; 0.5–6% incidence of pseudoaneurysm after femoral artery puncture
  - Popliteal aneurysm: bilateral in 50%; 33% of patients with popliteal aneurysm have AAA; usually asymptomatic; first symptoms often acute ischemia, thrombosis, peripheral embolization causing acute ischemia
  - Femoral aneurysm: throbbing mass in groin
  - Persistent sciatic artery aneurysm: painful, pulsatile buttock mass
  - Ultrasound confirms size, diagnosis, flow; arteriography is advised before operation

- **Differential Diagnosis**
  - Causes include degenerative, mycotic, mechanical, traumatic (post-instrumentation)

- **Treatment**
  - Popliteal artery aneurysm: exclude and bypass with saphenous vein
  - Femoral pseudoaneurysm: treat with ultrasound-guided compression

- **Pearl**

  Femoral pseudoaneurysm can be prevented by careful management of the arterial catheterization access site.

Reference

Diwan A et al: Incidence of femoral and popliteal aneurysms in patients with abdominal aortic aneurysms. J Vasc Surg 2003;31:863.

Arterial Occlusion, Acute

- ■ Essentials of Diagnosis
  - Sudden occlusion of previously patent artery supplying an extremity; caused by embolus, thrombosis, trauma, or dissection
  - Embolus: source is the heart in 85%
  - Thrombosis: occurs in hypercoagulable states, malignancy, or atherosclerotic vessel
  - Symptoms and signs include the "5 Ps": pain, pallor, pulselessness, paresthesias, paralysis; pallor followed by mottled cyanosis; if symptoms last >12 hours, unlikely to be salvageable

- ■ Differential Diagnosis
  - Thrombosis
  - Embolic events

- ■ Treatment
  - Embolism or thrombosis: immediate administration of heparin; arteriography can be diagnostic and sometimes therapeutic if no delay in treatment
  - Surgery: thrombolysis, surgical embolectomy (fastest to reestablish flow), arterial reconstruction in thrombotic event with atherosclerosis (alternative to thrombolytic therapy)
  - Compartment fasciotomies may be needed if ischemia is irreversible; fasciotomies required if ≥6 hours of complete ischemia to preserve remaining viable tissue
  - Prognosis: good if blood flow reestablished within 6 hours

- ■ Pearl

Remember the "5 Ps": pain, pallor, pulselessness, paresthesias, and paralysis.

Reference

Ouriel K et al: Acute lower limb ischemia: Determinants of outcome. Surgery 1998;124:336.

Arterial Trauma, Iatrogenic

- **Essentials of Diagnosis**
  - Traumatic pseudoaneurysm may result from arterial access for percutaneous catheter procedures; anticoagulation
  - Symptoms and signs include mass, which may be pulsating; bleeding; pain
  - Duplex ultrasound can identify ongoing leak, patency of vessel

- **Differential Diagnosis**
  - Distal ischemia
  - Embolus

- **Treatment**
  - Pseudoaneurysm usually resolves spontaneously; ultrasound-guided compression can be useful
  - Operative therapy includes primary repair of artery versus interposition graft
  - Surgery is indicated for distal ischemia, severe infection of pseudoaneurysm

- **Pearl**

Femoral pseudoaneurysm can be prevented by careful management of the arterial catheterization access site.

Reference

Hye RJ: Compression therapy for acute iatrogenic femoral pseudoaneurysms. Semin Vasc Surg 2000;13:58.

Arteriovenous Fistula

- **Essentials of Diagnosis**
  - Abnormal connection between artery and vein, congenital or acquired, located anywhere in body
  - Congenital: systemic effect is minimal; usually noted in infancy or childhood
  - Acquired: enlarges rapidly, can cause heart failure; continuous murmur may be heard; palpable thrill and increased skin temperature; proximal vein dilatation, diminished distal pulse, distal coolness
  - Magnetic resonance imaging (MRI) is study of choice for peripheral arteriovenous malformation; angiography precisely delineates arteriovenous fistula

- **Differential Diagnosis**
  - Systemic or distant intravascular infection

- **Treatment**
  - Monitor small peripheral fistulas
  - If treatment is needed, most are managed with radiographic embolization: head and neck, pelvis best
  - Operative management: ligate all feeding vessels

- **Pearl**

Small fistulas generally require no intervention.

Reference

White RI Jr et al: Long-term outcome of embolotherapy and surgery for high-flow extremity arteriovenous malformations. J Vasc Interv Radiol 2000; 11:1285.

Buerger Disease

- ■ Essentials of Diagnosis
    - • Also known as thromboangiitis obliterans; multiple segmental small artery occlusions in distal extremities; involves all 3 layers of arterial wall with infiltration of round cells
    - • Epidemiology: young cigarette-smoking men
    - • Symptoms and signs include migratory phlebitis; symptoms range from digital pain, to coolness and cyanosis, to necrosis and gangrene
    - • Angiography findings are distinctive but not pathognomonic; tapering of proximal vessels

- ■ Differential Diagnosis
    - • Precise diagnosis made only by microscopic evaluation

- ■ Treatment
    - • Cessation of smoking essential to avoid disease progression; disease may even become dormant
    - • Sympathectomy decreases arterial spasm in some patients
    - • Amputation for pain or gangrene
    - • Surgery is indicated for severe symptoms, necrosis, or gangrene

- ■ Pearl

Smoking cessation is critical to limit progression of disease.

Reference

Eichorn J et al: Antiendothelial cell antibodies in thromboangiitis obliterans. Am J Med 1998;315:17.

Carotid Aneurysm, Extracranial

- ■ Essentials of Diagnosis
  - • Rare, may occur anywhere along extracranial portion of carotid artery
  - • Symptoms and signs include pulsatile neck mass; dysphagia can occur from protrusion into oropharynx; neck pain, radiating to jaw; 30% present with transient ischemic attack (TIA)
  - • Duplex ultrasound is initial test; arteriography necessary to plan operation

- ■ Differential Diagnosis
  - • Rule out coiled or redundant carotid artery, subclavian artery (can present as pulsatile neck mass)

- ■ Treatment
  - • If accessible, resect and replace aneurysm with graft or vein; endovascular stenting may be an option
  - • Prognosis: good if reparable

- ■ Pearl

Evaluate for arterial aneurysms at other sites as well.

Reference

Rosset E et al: Surgical treatment of extracranial internal carotid artery aneurysms. J Vasc Surg 2000;31:713.

Carotid Body Tumor

- ■ Essentials of Diagnosis
  - • Carotid body: normally 3–6 mm; nest of chemoreceptor cells of neuroectodermal origin; responds to decrease in Po_2, increase in Pco_2, decrease in pH, or increase in blood temperature
  - • Tumors of carotid body: cervical chemodectomas, 10% metastatic; histologically, tumors resemble normal carotid body
  - • Symptoms and signs include slow enlargement of asymptomatic cervical mass; rarely, hypertension secondary to release of catecholamines; rarely, cranial nerve dysfunction from tumor extension; mass mobile in horizontal plane but not vertical plane
  - • Duplex ultrasound is often diagnostic

- ■ Differential Diagnosis
  - • Metastatic nodes from squamous cell cancer
  - • Thyroid cancer
  - • Carotid aneurysm

- ■ Treatment
  - • Preferred treatment is complete excision and arterial reconstruction if possible
  - • Complications: >50% incidence of cranial nerve dysfunction after resection

- ■ Pearl

Carotid body tumors are extremely vascular and require meticulous technique during resection.

Reference

Westerband A et al: Current trends in the detection and management of carotid body tumors. J Vasc Surg 1998;28:84.

Cerebrovascular Disease, Atherosclerotic

- **Essentials of Diagnosis**
  - Symptoms result more often from emboli than from hypoperfusion; 80% of patients with occlusive cerebrovascular disease have accessible arterial lesion in neck or chest; most strokes due to lesions of internal carotid, but can be from innominate artery or aorta
  - Symptoms and signs: in asymptomatic disease, bruit may be heard; in TIA, short-lived paresis or numbness of contralateral arm or leg that lasts <24 hours
  - Amaurosis fugax: microembolus to ophthalmic artery produces temporary mononuclear vision loss
  - Acute unstable neurologic defect: patients may have crescendo TIA, stroke in evolution, waxing and waning deficits
  - Completed stroke: 50% will suffer another stroke
  - Vertebrobasilar disease: emboli or hypoperfusion of posterior system causes drop attacks, clumsiness, vertigo, diplopia, dysphagia, disequilibrium
  - Carotid duplex ultrasound allows screening for stenosis; cerebral arteriography shows extracranial and intracranial anatomy of carotid and vertebral arteries

- **Differential Diagnosis**
  - Cardiac source of emboli

- **Treatment**
  - Objective is to prevent TIAs and strokes; all patients need aspirin, risk factor reduction, smoking cessation
  - Endarterectomy preferred for lesions of internal carotid, right vertebral, and right subclavian arteries
  - Surgery is indicated in asymptomatic patients if 80–99% stenosis on duplex ultrasound
  - Medications: aspirin, low-density lipoprotein–lowering agents, hypertension treatment
  - Prognosis: mortality from initial stroke is 20–30%; antiplatelet therapy deceases stroke rate by 5%

- **Pearl**

The stroke rate after endarterectomy must be kept low by expert surgeons for prophylactic intervention to be useful.

Reference

Ferguson GG et al: The North American Symptomatic Carotid Endarterectomy Trial: Surgical results in 1415 patients. Stroke 1999;30:1751.

Cerebrovascular Disease, Nonatherosclerotic

- ■ Essentials of Diagnosis
  - Takayasu arteritis: obliterative arteriopathy involving aortic arch vessels
  - Fibromuscular dysplasia: nonatherosclerotic angiopathy, unknown cause; affects specific arteries, usually bilateral disease; involves middle third of internal carotid
  - Symptoms and signs: internal carotid dissection: ipsilateral cerebral ischemic symptoms, acute neck pain, cervical tenderness at angle of mandible; fibromuscular dysplasia: 20% have had stroke at presentation
  - Imaging: for internal carotid dissection, duplex ultrasound indicates narrowing; arteriography shows characteristic tapered narrowing; if lumen persists, it resumes normal caliber beyond bony foramen; for fibromuscular dysplasia, arteriography shows characteristic "string of beads" appearance

- ■ Differential Diagnosis
  - Atherosclerotic cerebral disease
  - Takayasu arteritis
  - Dissecting aortic aneurysm
  - Internal carotid dissection
  - Fibromuscular dysplasia

- ■ Treatment
  - Takayasu arteritis: corticosteroids and cyclophosphamide
  - Internal carotid dissection: anticoagulation is treatment of choice; operation only for recurrent TIAs

- ■ Pearl

These are rare diseases, and prevention of permanent neurologic damage is the main goal of therapy.

Reference

Diwan A et al: Incidence of femoral and popliteal aneurysms in patients with abdominal aortic aneurysms. J Vasc Surg 2000;31:863.

Iliac Aneurysms

- ■ Essentials of Diagnosis
  - Occur with AAA in 20% of cases; rupture occurs but believed to be rare in aneurysms <3 cm
  - Symptoms and signs: 50% of patients are symptomatic, with compression or erosion into surrounding structures; rupture; erosion or rupture into ureter or bladder can cause hematuria, possibly massive
  - Workup: most symptomatic iliac aneurysms palpable on abdominal or rectal examination; perianal ecchymosis and decreased sphincter tone if pelvic or extraperitoneal rupture
  - Ultrasound, CT scan, MRI, or arteriography can diagnose

- ■ Differential Diagnosis
  - Causes include degenerative, mycotic, mechanical, traumatic (post-instrumentation)

- ■ Treatment
  - Solitary aneurysm: retroperitoneal approach is useful; hypogastric artery can be safely ligated if contralateral artery is normal
  - Bilateral common iliac artery aneurysm: bifurcated interposition graft
  - Currently, many are treated by endovascular repair

- ■ Pearl

Always evaluate for aneurysms at other sites.

Reference

Parsons RE et al: Midterm results of endovascular stented grafts for the treatment of isolated iliac artery aneurysms. J Vasc Surg 1999;30:915.

Intestinal Ischemia, Nonocclusive

- ■ Essentials of Diagnosis
  - No embolic or thrombotic cause of vascular obstruction; usually an associated low-flow state (sepsis, cardiac dysrhythmia)
  - Symptoms and signs include severe, poorly localized abdominal pain, often out of proportion to physical findings; nausea and vomiting; diarrhea; shock; gastrointestinal (GI) bleeding; abdominal distention; abdominal tenderness; peritonitis
  - Laboratory tests demonstrate leukocytosis, elevated serum amylase, significant base deficit
  - Abdominal x-ray is nonspecific; CT scan shows diffuse distention with air-fluid levels, intestinal wall thickening, intramural gas in portal venous system; arteriography documents absence of major vascular occlusion but otherwise not diagnostic in most cases

- ■ Differential Diagnosis
  - Intestinal ischemia due to embolic or thrombotic process
  - Acute pancreatitis
  - Intestinal obstruction

- ■ Treatment
  - Correct the cause of the low-flow state
  - Resect all necrotic bowel; perform second-look operation 12–24 hours later if marginally viable bowel was left; vascular reconstruction is ineffective
  - Surgery is indicated for suspected mesenteric ischemia
  - Complications: short gut syndrome, sepsis, multi-organ failure, death
  - Prognosis: mortality rate is near 90%, often because of underlying disease

- ■ Pearl

Avoid performing primary anastomosis.

Reference

Inderbitzi R et al: Acute mesenteric ischemia. Eur J Surg 1992;158:123.

Mesenteric Ischemia

- ■ Essentials of Diagnosis
  - • Chronic mesenteric ischemia: "intestinal angina"; results in ischemia upon "stressing" the gut with food intake
  - • Acute mesenteric ischemia: either embolic or thrombotic; due to embolus most often in superior mesenteric artery (SMA)
  - • Symptoms and signs: chronic mesenteric ischemia causes pain 15–30 minutes after eating; epigastric pain, radiating to upper quadrants; weight loss with fear of eating; epigastric bruit in 80%; pain out of proportion to physical examination findings
  - • Arteriography in anteroposterior and lateral views necessary; patients should be well hydrated to limit risk of hypercoagulability, decreased mesenteric blood flow, bowel infarction

- ■ Differential Diagnosis
  - • Peptic ulcer disease
  - • Gastroesophageal reflux disease
  - • Cholecystitis

- ■ Treatment
  - • Chronic mesenteric ischemia; atherosclerotic lesion: surgical revascularization by endarterectomy or bypass
  - • Acute mesenteric ischemia: identify occluded vessel; perform arteriotomy, embolectomy with catheter, or may need bypass; if bowel not viable, bowel resection
  - • Median arcuate ligament syndrome: divide ligament with or without arterial bypass
  - • Surgery is indicated for acute mesenteric ischemia, chronic symptomatic ischemia with flow-limiting lesion(s)

- ■ Pearl

Magnetic resonance angiography may be diagnostic and less likely than arteriography to cause dehydration and mesenteric thrombosis.

Reference

Kazmers A: Operative management of chronic mesenteric ischemia. Ann Vasc Surg 1998;12:299.

Mesenteric Vascular Occlusion, Acute

- ■ Essentials of Diagnosis
  - Causes include mesenteric arterial emboli (50%); thrombosis of a mesenteric artery (25%); rarely, dissecting aortic aneurysm, connective tissue disorders, cocaine ingestion
  - Symptoms and signs include severe, poorly localized abdominal pain that is often out of proportion to physical findings; nausea and vomiting; diarrhea; shock; GI bleeding; abdominal distention; abdominal tenderness; peritonitis
  - Laboratory tests show leukocytosis, significant base deficit
  - Abdominal x-ray is nonspecific; specific findings occur late; CT scan shows diffuse distention with air-fluid levels, intestinal wall thickening, intramural gas, gas in portal venous system

- ■ Differential Diagnosis
  - Acute pancreatitis
  - Strangulation obstruction
  - Nonocclusive intestinal ischemia

- ■ Treatment
  - Resection of all involved gut; revascularization of proximal stenosis to salvage viable bowel
  - Thrombectomy usually unsuccessful; role of angioplasty not yet defined
  - Treatment monitoring: second-look operation is performed 12–24 hours after initial operation if marginally viable bowel was left
  - Prognosis: mortality rate with arterial occlusion, 45%; with venous thrombosis, 30%; repeat thrombosis 25% without warfarin

- ■ Pearl

A prospectively planned second-look operation can help to preserve bowel length.

Reference

Boley SJ, Brandt LJ: Intestinal ischemia. Surg Clin North Am 1992;72:1.

Popliteal Artery Diseases

- **Essentials of Diagnosis**
  - Popliteal entrapment: rare cause of stenosis or occlusion; occurs because of anomalous course of popliteal artery; popliteal artery passes medially to medial head of gastrocnemius muscle (normally passes laterally)
  - Cystic degeneration of popliteal artery: arterial stenosis produced by mucoid cyst in adventitia; located in middle third of artery
  - Symptoms and signs of popliteal entrapment range from calf claudication to severe ischemia; cystic degeneration of popliteal artery causes calf claudication most commonly; decreased pedal pulse strength; mass may be palpated (rarely)
  - Imaging: for popliteal artery entrapment, MRI often useful for diagnosis; for cystic degeneration of popliteal artery, arteriography localizes zone of popliteal stenosis; ultrasound or CT scan can demonstrate cyst in artery wall

- **Differential Diagnosis**
  - Popliteal aneurysm
  - Atherosclerotic disease

- **Treatment**
  - Popliteal entrapment: division of medial head of gastrocnemius muscle; graft replacement of diseased artery
  - Cystic degeneration of popliteal artery: cyst excision, although may recur; arterial excision and graft replacement necessary in some patients

- **Pearl**

Always evaluate the popliteal artery in patients with foot symptoms.

Reference

O'Hara N et al: Surgical treatment for popliteal artery entrapment syndrome. Cardiovasc Surg 2001;9:141.

Renal Artery Aneurysms

- ■ Essentials of Diagnosis
    - • Uncommon; occur in <0.1% of population; associated with hypertension; occur slightly more often in women than in men
    - • Usually saccular and located at primary or secondary bifurcation; 4 categories: true aneurysm, dissecting aneurysm, aneurysm associated with fibrodysplastic disease, arteritis-related microaneurysm
    - • Renovascular hypertension can be due to associated arterial stenosis, dissection, arteriovenous fistula, thromboembolism
    - • Rupture is rare except during pregnancy
    - • Symptoms and signs: most cases are asymptomatic; discovered incidentally or during workup for hypertension
    - • Angiography or MRI for definition

- ■ Differential Diagnosis
    - • Consider arteritis
    - • Evaluate other sites of aneurysm formation (visceral and peripheral)

- ■ Treatment
    - • Small renal aneurysms are followed conservatively with CT scans, angiography every 2 years
    - • Surgery: repair in situ or ligate and bypass; nephrectomy is necessary if aneurysm has ruptured
    - • Surgery is indicated for women of childbearing age, patients with associated renal artery disease, large aneurysms (increased rate of rupture with larger aneurysms not proven)

- ■ Pearl

Always evaluate for other sites of aneurysms.

Reference

Messina LM et al: Visceral artery aneurysms. Surg Clin North Am 1997;77:425.

Renovascular Hypertension

- ■ Essentials of Diagnosis
  - • Usually caused by renal artery stenosis: 67% caused by atherosclerosis; 33% fibromuscular dysplasia
  - • Fibromuscular dysplasia: involves middle to distal 33% of renal artery; medial dysplasia most common (85%); 2–7% of hypertension is caused by renovascular disease
  - • Symptoms and signs: most patients are asymptomatic or have irritability, headache, depression; persistent elevation of diastolic blood pressure; bruit frequently present in abdomen
  - • Selective renal vein renin levels: renal vein renin ratio of involved kidney to uninvolved kidney >1.5 is diagnostic
  - • Intravenous pyelography is common screening test to compare kidneys; atrophic kidney suggests diagnosis; renal arteriography is most precise for delineating obstructive lesion; duplex ultrasound is up to 90% sensitive

- ■ Differential Diagnosis
  - • Essential hypertension
  - • Aortic coarctation
  - • Hyperaldosteronism
  - • Cushing disease
  - • Pheochromocytoma

- ■ Treatment
  - • Primarily treated with medical therapy, angioplasty, or both
  - • Endarterectomy if lesion is focal and close to aorta
  - • Arterial replacement preferred for fibromuscular dysplasia
  - • Nephrectomy should be considered if unilateral atrophic kidney
  - • Prognosis: percutaneous transluminal angioplasty shows 90% immediate success in patients with fibromuscular dysplasia

- ■ Pearl

Screening is necessary to detect this cause of hypertension.

Reference

Helin KH et al: Predicting the outcome of invasive treatment of renal artery disease. J Intern Med 2000;247:105.

Superior Mesenteric Artery Obstruction of the Duodenum

- ■ Essentials of Diagnosis
  - Obstruction of the third portion of duodenum by compression between superior mesenteric vessels and aorta; usually appears after rapid weight loss following injury or burns
  - Symptoms and signs include epigastric bloating, crampy pain relieved by vomiting; symptoms may remit in the prone position; anorexia and postprandial pain lead to additional malnutrition and weight loss
  - Upper GI contrast radiography is diagnostic; angiography shows angle of ≤25 degrees between SMA and aorta

- ■ Differential Diagnosis
  - Intestinal malrotation with duodenal obstruction by congenital bands
  - Involvement of duodenum by scleroderma with diminished peristalsis

- ■ Treatment
  - Postural therapy may suffice: patient should be prone in knee-chest position when symptomatic or when anticipating postprandial difficulties
  - Surgery: for chronic obstruction, division of suspensory ligament and mobilization of duodenum, or duodenojejunostomy; for malrotation, mobilization of duodenojejunal flexure

- ■ Pearl

Symptoms may be subtle and difficult to diagnose in patients with an initiating cause for weight loss.

Reference

Diwakaran HH et al: Superior mesenteric artery syndrome. Gastroenterology 2001;121:516,746.

Thoracic Aortic Aneurysms

■ Essentials of Diagnosis

- Can be saccular or fusiform; common causes include atherosclerosis, medial degeneration of aortic wall, Marfan syndrome (defect in fibrillin gene)
- Symptoms and signs, if present, are due to local pressure or obstruction of adjacent structures; ascending aorta: aortic regurgitation, superior vena cava obstruction, chest pain; aortic arch: tracheal compression; descending aorta: recurrent laryngeal nerve compression, phrenic paralysis, dysphagia, stridor
- Chest film may show convex right cardiac border in ascending aneurysms, prominent aortic knob in arch aneurysms, posterior lateral thoracic mass in descending aneurysms; CT scan or magnetic resonance angiography may define anatomy and extent of aneurysm

■ Differential Diagnosis

- Mediastinal tumor

■ Treatment

- Primary determinants for repair: aneurysm size, cause, and symptoms
- Asymptomatic aneurysms measuring ≤5.5 cm: aggressive blood pressure control with β-blockers
- Aneurysms measuring >5.5 cm: consider repair, especially if symptoms are present
- Complications: spinal cord ischemia in descending aortic repair, 5–15%
- Prognosis: operative mortality, 5–15%; 10-year survival for ascending, 50%; descending, 38%

■ Pearl

Morbidity and mortality of repair are significantly greater than those for AAA.

Reference

Coady MA et al: Natural history, pathogenesis, and etiology of thoracic aortic aneurysms and dissections. Cardiol Clin 1999;17:615.

Thoracic Aortic Dissection

- ■ Essentials of Diagnosis
  - Often lethal event; degeneration of aortic media is hallmark of disease; location of intimal tear: ascending aorta, 62%; arch, 10%; isthmus, 16%; rest in distal aorta
  - Classification: DeBakey type I originates in ascending aorta, extends beyond left subclavian (Stanford type A); DeBakey type II involves ascending aorta only, associated with aortic valve incompetence (Stanford type A); DeBakey type III occurs distal to left subclavian artery, often extends into abdominal aorta (Stanford type B)
  - Symptoms and signs: most common is severe, tearing chest pain, often signifies intimal tear and formation of false lumen; ascending aorta: pain is anterior; descending aorta: pain is posterior between scapulas; hypotension with blood loss, leak into pericardium; sudden death if extension into pericardium or down a coronary artery; if aortic valve or root involved, aortic insufficiency and acute congestive heart failure
  - Chest film shows widened mediastinum in 50%; chest CT is diagnostic procedure of choice; transesophageal echocardiography is diagnostic; gives information about myocardial function, aortic valve competence

- ■ Differential Diagnosis
  - Myocardial infarction
  - Pulmonary embolism
  - Gastroesophageal reflux disease

- ■ Treatment
  - Immediate and effective blood pressure control is critical; esmolol commonly used (decreases dP/dT and aortic shear force)
  - Medications: β-blockers (esmolol); vasodilators if still hypertensive after β-blockade
  - Angiographic fenestration or operative repair is high risk; must revascularize vital organs
  - Prognosis: for repair of ascending aorta, operative mortality is 5%; 5-year survival, 55%; for emergent repair of descending aorta, operative mortality is 15%

- ■ Pearl
  Blood pressure control is critical.

Reference

Sabik JF et al: Long-term effectiveness of operations for ascending aortic dissections. J Thorac Cardiovasc Surg 2000;119:946.

Thoracic Outlet Syndrome

- **Essentials of Diagnosis**
  - Variety of disorders caused by arterial, venous, or nerve compression at base of neck
  - Symptoms and signs are predominantly neurologic; pain, paresthesias, numbness in brachial plexus trunks (ulnar most common); hand numbness often wakes patients from sleep; motor deficits indicate long duration
  - Adson test: weakened radial pulse with arm abduction and head rotated to opposite side
  - Tinel sign: light percussion in supraclavicular fossa produces peripheral sensations
  - Subclavian artery compression: bruit, distal emboli, or arterial occlusion
  - Subclavian vein compression: thrombosis of vein leading to extremity pain and swelling (effort thrombosis called Paget-von Schrötter syndrome)

- **Differential Diagnosis**
  - Carpal tunnel syndrome
  - Cervical disk disease

- **Treatment**
  - Postural correction and physical therapy
  - If surgical repair warranted, thoracic outlet decompression; 2 approaches possible: supraclavicular, transaxillary
  - Surgery is indicated for arterial disease, venous compression, neurologic symptoms not attributable to other disease, failure of conservative therapy after 3–6 months

- **Pearl**

Clinical judgment is critical to choose patients who may benefit from operative decompression.

Reference

Sharp WJ et al: Long-term follow-up and patient satisfaction after surgery for thoracic outlet syndrome. Ann Vasc Surg 2001;15:32.

Vascular Occlusive Disease, Peripheral

- ### Essentials of Diagnosis
  - Predominantly affects lower extremities
  - Symptoms and signs include intermittent claudication: pain, fatigue, cramping in leg muscles (most often calf) with walking; relieved by 2–5 minutes of rest
  - Ischemic rest pain: severe, burning pain in forefoot aggravated by leg elevation, improved with leg in dependent position
  - Nonhealing wound ulcers: trivial trauma may cause wounds
  - Leriche syndrome (aortoiliac disease): claudication of hip, thigh, buttock; atrophy of leg muscles; impotence; diminished femoral pulses
  - Color duplex ultrasound can identify arterial lesions but is operator dependent; arteriography provides anatomic location of disease; magnetic resonance angiography can delineate arteries without contrast, but overestimates disease

- ### Differential Diagnosis
  - Osteoarthritis
  - Neurospinal compression (spinal stenosis)
  - Venous claudication
  - Vasculitis
  - Aortic coarctation
  - Popliteal entrapment, popliteal cysts
  - Persistent sciatic arteries
  - External iliac dysplasias
  - Primary vascular tumors
  - Diabetic neuropathy pain

- ### Treatment
  - Objectives are symptom relief and limb salvage
  - Risk reduction: stop smoking, control blood pressure, lower cholesterol (low-density lipoprotein goal <100 mg/dL), control diabetes, exercise to increase claudication distance
  - β-Blockers before surgery if patient tolerates
  - Bypass or endarterectomy for diseased segment
  - Prognosis: without diabetes, 5-year survival 70%; with cerebrovascular or ischemic heart disease, 5-year survival 60%; with renal failure, 2-year survival <50%

- ### Pearl

Occlusive vascular disease is a systemic illness; always evaluate for cardiac or cerebrovascular effects.

Reference

Donnelly R et al: ABC of arterial and venous disease: Vascular complications of diabetes. BMJ 2000;320:1062.

Vasoconstrictive Disorders

■ Essentials of Diagnosis

- Raynaud syndrome: precipitated by exposure to cold or stress; may follow virulent or benign course
- Acrocyanosis: persistent cyanosis of hands and feet; occurs in young females
- Scleroderma: connective tissue disease; fibrosis due to increased collagen and elastin, arterial intimal thickening
- Reflex sympathetic dystrophy: post-traumatic pain syndrome, poorly understood
- Symptoms and signs: Raynaud syndrome causes sequence of pallor, cyanosis, rubor (white-blue-red color changes); acrocyanosis causes cyanosis, numbness, and pain; changes disappear when warm; scleroderma first affects skin and vasculature of hands; skin is thick and taut, with limited finger flexion; reflex sympathetic dystrophy causes exquisite pain to minimal stimuli, progressive muscle atrophy

■ Differential Diagnosis

- Occlusive vascular disease
- Chronic emboli

■ Treatment

- Raynaud syndrome and acrocyanosis: avoid cold, tobacco, oral contraceptives, and β-blockers; calcium channel blockers, prostaglandins, ketanserin, oral papaverine may be helpful
- Scleroderma: palliative treatment; sympathectomy rarely helps; corticosteroids slow progression
- Reflex sympathetic dystrophy: sympathetic block; surgical sympathectomy; spinal cord stimulation; intrathecal baclofen gives temporary pain relief

■ Pearl

Always evaluate for occlusive or embolic disease.

Reference

Schwartzman RJ: New treatments for reflex sympathetic dystrophy. N Engl J Med 2000;343:654.

Visceral Aneurysms

- **Essentials of Diagnosis**
  - Include splenic, hepatic, and SMA aneurysms
  - Splenic artery aneurysm: ruptures in <2%, rarely if <3 cm
  - Hepatic artery aneurysm: 20% rupture frequency
  - SMA aneurysm: aneurysm may involve origin or branches of SMA
  - Symptoms and signs: splenic artery aneurysm often asymptomatic, occasionally abdominal pain, rupture; hepatic artery aneurysm ruptures into peritoneal cavity, biliary tree, or viscus; hemobilia occurs with rupture into biliary tree; 33% of patients have triad of intermittent abdominal pain, GI bleeding, jaundice; SMA aneurysm causes nonspecific abdominal pain, mobile pulsatile abdominal mass, abdominal apoplexy with rupture
  - Imaging: in splenic artery aneurysm, abdominal x-ray shows concentric calcification in left upper quadrant; CT scan and angiogram often diagnostic; in hepatic artery or SMA aneurysm, CT scan helpful

- **Differential Diagnosis**
  - Other causes of abdominal pain or mass
  - AAA

- **Treatment**
  - Splenic artery aneurysm: surgery is indicated for symptomatic aneurysm, pregnant women with aneurysm, any aneurysm >3 cm
  - Hepatic artery aneurysm and SMA aneurysm: surgery is indicated for rupture, pain, or other local compressive effects

- **Pearl**

Evaluate for other sites of aneurysm.

Reference

Carr SC et al: Visceral artery aneurysm rupture. J Vasc Surg 2001;33:806.

13

Veins & Lymphatics

Deep Venous Thrombosis

- **Essentials of Diagnosis**
  - Virchow triad: stasis, vascular injury, hypercoagulability
  - Symptoms and signs: 50% are asymptomatic; thigh or calf pain with or without edema; extensive deep venous thrombosis (DVT) causes massive edema, cyanosis, dilated superficial veins, low-grade fever, tachycardia; 50% have positive Homans sign (calf pain with ankle dorsiflexion); acute pulmonary embolism (PE); phlegmasia
  - Duplex ultrasound has sensitivity and specificity >95%; magnetic resonance venography has sensitivity and specificity nearly 100%

- **Differential Diagnosis**
  - Local muscle strain; Achilles tendon rupture
  - Cellulitis; lymphedema
  - Baker cyst obstructing popliteal vein; retroperitoneal mass obstructing iliac vein
  - Congestive heart failure
  - Liver or kidney failure
  - Inferior vena cava (IVC) obstruction

- **Treatment**
  - Goal is to reduce complications
  - Anticoagulation: decreases recurrence and PE risk by 80%; limits propagation of clot (no effect on clot lysis)
  - Surgery is indicated for calf compartment syndrome; massive extremity edema
  - Medications: heparin potentiates antithrombin III, inhibits thrombin; warfarin is initiated when partial thromboplastin time therapeutic; in first few days, may be hypercoagulable from inhibition of anticoagulant proteins C and S; low-molecular-weight heparin inhibits factor Xa activity; lower risk of bleeding
  - IVC filter placement may be beneficial for patients with contraindications to anticoagulation and ongoing risk of thromboembolism

- **Pearl**

Most DVT is asymptomatic.

Reference

Hirsh J et al: Clinical trials that have influenced the treatment of venous thromboembolism: A historical perspective. Ann Intern Med 2001;134:409.

Deep Venous Thrombosis, Upper Extremity

- ■ Essentials of Diagnosis
  - • Axillary-subclavian thrombosis: 3 causes: Paget-von Schrötter syndrome, also called "effort thrombosis," from intermittent obstruction of vein during repetitive arm or shoulder movements; primary subclavian venous thrombosis occurs in patients with hypercoagulable states; secondary subclavian venous thrombosis results from venous injury (central lines, external trauma, pacemaker wires)
  - • Symptoms and signs: Paget-von Schrötter causes significant superficial venous distention in arm or shoulder; aching pain; cyanosis of chest wall, axilla, shoulder, and arm; subclavian venous thrombosis causes edematous, cyanotic arm and hand
  - • Perform duplex ultrasound of upper extremity; consider venography and thrombolysis if duplex ultrasound is abnormal

- ■ Differential Diagnosis
  - • Evaluate for other evidence of hypercoagulability

- ■ Treatment
  - • Remove indwelling central lines or pacemakers; elevate arm; hydrate with intravenous (IV) fluid
  - • Vein compression with large collaterals suggests venous thoracic outlet syndrome and necessitates early operation

- ■ Pearl

Most upper-extremity DVT is asymptomatic.

Reference

Urschel HC et al: Paget-Schroetter syndrome: What is the best management? Ann Thorac Surg 2000;69:1663.

Lymphedema & Lymphangitis

- **Essentials of Diagnosis**
  - Lymphedema: little is known about fluid dynamics of lymphatic system; lymph propulsion occurs from lymphatic smooth muscle contractions; 2–4 L/d drains into subclavian vein
  - Primary disease is due to abnormal lymphatic development; secondary disease is due to obstruction of lymphatic system; most common cause is surgical excision, also radiation to axillary or inguinal areas
  - Lymphangitis: caused by hemolytic *Streptococcus* or *Staphylococcus* infection in area of cellulitis near open wound; multiple long red streaks are seen coursing toward lymph nodes
  - Symptoms and signs: lymphedema is slowly progressive and painless; in early stages, edema is pitting; with time, fibrosis occurs and edema becomes non-pitting; centered around ankle, pronounced around dorsum of foot and toes; thickened skin, hyperkeratosis; lymphangitis causes pain at wound site, often red streaks along lymphatics toward lymph nodes, regional lymph node enlargement
  - Imaging: for lymphedema, venous duplex ultrasound excludes venous insufficiency; lymphangiography is rarely useful

- **Differential Diagnosis**
  - Congestive heart failure
  - Chronic renal insufficiency; chronic hepatic insufficiency; chronic venous insufficiency
  - Congenital vascular malformations
  - Reflex sympathetic dystrophy
  - Lymphangitis: superficial thrombophlebitis, cat-scratch fever, cellulitis

- **Treatment**
  - Lymphedema: no cure; goal of therapy is to reduce complications; pneumatic compression is first-line therapy
  - Lymphangitis: elevate extremity; apply warm compresses; administer IV antibiotics

- **Pearl**

Cellulitis in an extremity with lymphedema can be difficult to eradicate.

Reference

Pain SJ et al: Lymphoedema following surgery for breast cancer. Br J Surg 2000;87:1128.

Pulmonary Thromboembolism

- ■ Essentials of Diagnosis
  - • DVT is most common source of PE; <10% of PE cases cause pulmonary infarction
  - • Symptoms and signs include dyspnea and chest pain (present in 75%); tachycardia, tachypnea, altered mental status; classic triad of dyspnea, chest pain, and hemoptysis in only 15%; pleural rub and S1Q3T3 rarely found
  - • V̇/Q̇ scan has sensitivity and specificity of 90%, but 67% of studies are inconclusive; spiral computed tomography is more accurate

- ■ Differential Diagnosis
  - • Other causes of chest pain and hypoxia, such as pneumonia

- ■ Treatment
  - • Stabilize initially with pressors and ventilatory support; start heparin or low-molecular-weight heparin quickly
  - • Surgery: consider IVC filter if risk of embolus is ongoing and anti-coagulation is risky
  - • Open surgical thrombectomy (Trendelenburg procedure): high mortality, rarely clinically useful for massive saddle embolus
  - • Prevention: DVT prophylaxis in perioperative period

- ■ Pearl

Pulmonary embolism is the initial symptom in many patients with DVT.

Reference

Cross JJ et al: A randomized trial of spiral CT and ventilation perfusion scintigraphy for the diagnosis of pulmonary embolism. Clin Radiol 1998;53:177.

Thrombophlebitis, Superficial

- ■ Essentials of Diagnosis
  - • Can occur spontaneously in varicose veins, pregnant or postpartum women, thromboangiitis obliterans, Behçet disease; superficial migratory phlebitis (Trousseau) suggests abdominal carcinoma
  - • Symptoms and signs include local extremity pain, redness; indurated, erythematous, tender areas indicate thrombosed superficial veins; well localized over superficial vein

- ■ Differential Diagnosis
  - • Ascending lymphangitis
  - • Cellulitis
  - • Erythema nodosum
  - • Erythema induration
  - • Panniculitis

- ■ Treatment
  - • Primary treatment includes nonsteroidal anti-inflammatory drugs, heat, elevation, support stockings, elastic wrap; ambulation is encouraged
  - • Surgery: excise vein if condition persists >2 weeks or recurs; ligate and resect vein at saphenofemoral or cephalic-subclavian junction
  - • Prognosis: uncomplicated superficial thrombophlebitis responds well to conservative therapy; extension into DVT may be associated with PE

- ■ Pearl

Always search for an underlying illness in patients with superficial thrombophlebitis.

Reference

Belcaro G et al: Superficial thrombophlebitis of the legs: A randomized, controlled, follow-up study. Angiology 1999;50:523.

Varicose Veins

- ■ Essentials of Diagnosis
  - Dilated, tortuous superficial veins in lower extremities, usually bilateral; due to genetic or developmental defects in vein wall causing valvular incompetence; most cases of isolated superficial venous insufficiency are primary
  - Symptoms and signs: many patients are asymptomatic or have localized pain (ache or heaviness with prolonged standing), phlebitis
  - Predominantly located medially (saphenous vein); Brodie-Trendelenburg test identifies saphenofemoral dysfunction

- ■ Differential Diagnosis
  - Chronic deep venous insufficiency
  - Klippel-Trenaunay syndrome: varicose veins, unilateral limb hypertrophy, and cutaneous birthmark (port wine stain; venous malformation)

- ■ Treatment
  - First manage venous insufficiency: elastic stockings, leg elevation, exercise; avoid prolonged sitting or standing
  - Surgical options: remove entire saphenous vein for incompetent saphenofemoral junction, varicosities along entire length; selective varicose vein removal with stab-avulsion technique for persistent or disabling pain, recurrent superficial thrombophlebitis, erosion of overlying skin with bleeding
  - Prognosis: 10% recurrence after treatment

- ■ Pearl

For most patients, venous varicosity disease is a cosmetic problem only, but for some, it is quite disabling.

Reference

Belcaro G et al: Endovascular sclerotherapy, surgery, and surgery plus sclerotherapy in superficial venous incompetence: A randomized, 10 year follow-up trial—final results. Angiology 2000;51:529.

Venous Insufficiency, Chronic

- **Essentials of Diagnosis**
  - Caused by chronic elevation in venous pressure; 3 factors: calf muscle pump dysfunction, valvular reflux, outflow obstruction
  - Symptoms and signs: first symptom usually ankle and calf edema, worse at end of day, improves with leg elevation; involvement of foot and toes suggests lymphedema; long-lasting disease causes stasis dermatitis, hyperpigmentation, brawny induration
  - Duplex ultrasound can locate incompetent perforating veins, but does not assess calf muscle function or proximal obstruction; venography determines functional outflow obstruction; descending phlebography tests valves and identifies reflux

- **Differential Diagnosis**
  - Lymphedema: nonpitting edema of foot and toes
  - Acute DVT
  - Congestive heart failure
  - Chronic liver disease; chronic kidney disease
  - Arterial insufficiency: ulcer is more distal and painful
  - Erythema nodosum
  - Fungal infections

- **Treatment**
  - Disease is incurable
  - Antireflux procedures include perforating vein ligation for incompetent perforating veins
  - Bypass operations for obstruction include Palma procedure: cross-femoral bypass with contralateral proximal saphenous vein; can use prosthetic material
  - Angioplasty and stenting for May-Thurner syndrome
  - Surgery is indicated for nonhealing ulcers; disabling symptoms

- **Pearl**

Lower-extremity venous stasis can be a severe, disabling disease.

Reference

Mohr DN et al: The venous stasis syndrome after deep venous thrombosis or pulmonary embolism: A population-based study. Mayo Clin Proc 2000;75:1249.

Section IV

Upper Gastrointestinal Surgery

Chapters

14

Esophagus & Diaphragm

Achalasia

- **Essentials of Diagnosis**
  - Neuromuscular disorder of esophageal dilation and hypertrophy without organic stenosis; cause is unknown, but 2 theories include degenerative disease of neurons or infection of neurons by a virus (eg, herpes zoster) or other pathogen
  - Symptoms and signs: dysphagia is dominant symptom; weight loss is not usually marked despite functional obstruction; pain is infrequent; regurgitation of retained esophageal contents is common, especially while sleeping
  - Contrast radiography and endoscopy show narrowing at the cardia; dilated body of the esophagus blends into a smooth cone-shaped area of narrowing 3–6 cm long; on manometry, body of the esophagus lacks primary peristaltic waves, but pressure in the gastroesophageal sphincter is increased
  - Workup: perform contrast radiographic or endoscopic studies; endoscopy is essential for establishing the diagnosis and excluding other causes of symptoms; manometry is useful for confirming the diagnosis

- **Differential Diagnosis**
  - Benign strictures of lower esophagus
  - Carcinoma at or near cardioesophageal junction
  - Diffuse esophageal spasm

- **Treatment**
  - Goal is to relieve functional obstruction by either pneumatic dilation or longitudinal division of all esophageal muscular layers (Heller myotomy)
  - Surgery is indicated for advanced disease, failed dilation
  - Prognosis: for dilation, long-term results are good in only 50%; for surgery, results are good to excellent in 90% of patients

- **Pearl**

  Always rule out cancer with distal esophageal obstruction.

Reference

Finley RJ et al: Laparoscopic Heller myotomy improves esophageal emptying and the symptoms of achalasia. Arch Surg 2001;136:892.

Barrett Esophagus

- **Essentials of Diagnosis**
    - Metaplastic changes from squamous to intestinal-type columnar epithelium in the distal esophagus; metaplasia may contain varying degrees of dysplasia, which is associated with a 2-fold increased risk of esophageal adenocarcinoma; found in 10–20% of patients with gastroesophageal reflux disease (GERD)
    - Symptoms and signs include heartburn, milder than in the absence of Barrett changes because metaplastic epithelium is less sensitive than squamous epithelium; regurgitation; dysphagia
    - Esophagoscopy shows pink epithelium in lower esophagus instead of shiny gray-pink squamous mucosa; must be verified by biopsy
    - Workup: patients with moderate to severe GERD should undergo endoscopy and biopsy to assess distal esophagus for metaplastic changes; only biopsy-proven intestinal-type metaplasia is associated with increased risk of adenocarcinoma

- **Differential Diagnosis**
    - High-grade dysplasia
    - Adenocarcinoma

- **Treatment**
    - Treatment is the same as for GERD; surgical treatment is fundoplication
    - Surgery is indicated for severe GERD refractory to medical treatment; esophageal strictures and ulcers; esophagectomy for high-grade dysplasia
    - Medications: H_2-blocking agents, proton pump inhibitors, antacids
    - Monitor treatment with routine endoscopy and biopsy every 6–12 months to assess degree of dysplasia
    - Prognosis: metaplastic epithelium rarely regresses after medical or surgical therapy; estimated incidence of adenocarcinoma with Barrett esophagus is 1 in 100 patient-years of follow-up

- **Pearl**

Surveillance for carcinoma development is mandatory in patients with Barrett esophagus.

Reference

Spechler SJ et al: Long-term outcome of medical and surgical therapies for gastroesophageal reflux disease: Follow-up of a randomized controlled trial. JAMA 2001;285:2331.

Epiphrenic Diverticulum

- **Essentials of Diagnosis**
  - Usually located in distal 10 cm of the esophagus but may occur as high as the mid thorax; usually associated with uncoordinated smooth muscle activity in distal esophagus
  - Symptoms and signs include dysphagia, regurgitation, aspiration, spasm-type chest pain, heartburn
  - Contrast radiography shows contrast-filled smooth pouch in the distal esophagus, possible distal esophageal narrowing; manometry reveals simultaneous repetitive contractions in body of the esophagus
  - Workup: perform upper gastrointestinal (GI) contrast radiography with fluoroscopy; esophagoscopy; esophageal manometry in every case to evaluate underlying motility disorders and assess lower esophageal sphincter; pH monitoring may be added to further evaluate lower esophageal sphincter dysfunction and associated reflux

- **Differential Diagnosis**
  - Carcinoma
  - Benign strictures
  - Esophageal webs
  - Achalasia
  - Diffuse esophageal spasm

- **Treatment**
  - Diverticulectomy and longitudinal myotomy to include the lower esophageal sphincter, extending proximally to the level where esophageal function becomes normal on manometry
  - Surgery is indicated for moderate to severe symptoms
  - Prognosis: surgery is successful in 80–90% of cases

- **Pearl**

Beware of underlying motility disorders of the esophagus because operation may not produce the desired effects.

Reference

Thomas ML et al: Oesophageal diverticula. Br J Surg 2001;88:629.

Esophageal Carcinoma

- **Essentials of Diagnosis**
  - Represents 1% of all malignant lesions and 6% of GI tract cancers
  - Symptoms and signs include dysphagia; weight loss and weakness; difficulty swallowing solid foods initially, followed by both solids and liquids; pain that may be related to swallowing; regurgitation and aspiration; coughing related to swallowing; hoarseness that usually reflects spread to the recurrent laryngeal nerves
  - Barium swallow demonstrates narrowing of the lumen at site of the lesion and dilation proximally; tumor appears as an irregular mass; esophagoscopy with biopsy provides a tissue diagnosis in 95% of cases; endoscopic ultrasound shows wall penetration and mediastinal invasion; computed tomography (CT) scan shows distant mediastinal and celiac axis nodal metastases
  - Workup: perform barium swallow, esophagoscopy with biopsy, endoscopic ultrasound, CT scan; because lesions of the upper and mid esophagus may invade the tracheobronchial tree, bronchoscopy is always indicated to assess growths at these levels

- **Differential Diagnosis**
  - Benign strictures
  - Benign papillomas, polyps, or granular cell tumors

- **Treatment**
  - Preoperative radiation may convert unresectable tumor to a resectable one; about 50% of tumors are resectable at presentation and about 75% after radiotherapy and chemotherapy
  - Esophagectomy is indicated for cure or palliation in suitable candidates without distant metastases
  - Prognosis: 5-year survival after curative resection is about 30% for patients with squamous cell carcinoma and 10% for patients with adenocarcinoma

- **Pearl**

Operative resection alone has a substantial recurrence risk.

References

Lew JI et al: Long-term survival following induction chemoradiotherapy and esophagectomy for esophageal carcinoma. Arch Surg 2001;135:737.

National Comprehensive Cancer Network: Practice Guidelines. http://www.nccn.org

Esophageal Obstruction

■ **Essentials of Diagnosis**
- Causes include ingestion of foreign object or bolus of meat; esophageal bands or webs
- Foreign objects usually lodge just beyond the cricopharyngeus
- Bands or webs may develop at any level but are most frequent in the subcricoid region; Schatzki ring is a narrow mucosal ring at the squamocolumnar junction; may be asymptomatic or cause dysphagia, chest pain, respiratory distress
- Endoscopy will identify foreign objects suspected of causing esophageal obstruction; endoscopy or contrast radiography may identify esophageal rings, bands, or webs that may be associated with esophagitis

■ **Differential Diagnosis**
- Underlying esophageal disease precipitating obstruction, particularly with meat impaction

■ **Treatment**
- Foreign objects: 90% reach the stomach and pass without incident; 10% require endoscopic removal, including 1% requiring surgery; button batteries are highly corrosive and should be removed promptly
- Surgery is indicated for inability to treat endoscopically; all ingested packets containing cocaine
- Webs, rings, and bands: most are treated effectively by dilation
- Prognosis: 1500 deaths yearly from complications of ingested foreign bodies

■ **Pearl**

Perform endoscopy or contrast swallow early in management.

Reference

Arana A et al: Management of ingested foreign bodies in childhood and review of the literature. Eur J Pediatr 2001;160:468.

Esophageal Perforation

- ■ Essentials of Diagnosis
  - • Causes include instrumentation, severe vomiting, and external trauma; morbidity is principally due to infection; signs of mediastinal or thoracic sepsis occur within 24 hours; esophageal defect usually breaks down if it is closed
  - • Symptoms and signs: with cervical perforations, pain is followed by crepitus in the neck, dysphagia, and signs of infection; thoracic perforations cause tachypnea, hyperpnea, dyspnea, and hypotension
  - • Laboratory findings: thoracentesis reveals cloudy or purulent fluid
  - • Workup: perform esophagogram promptly using water-soluble contrast medium to confirm level and extent of injury

- ■ Differential Diagnosis
  - • Rule out coexistent esophageal carcinoma, in which case treatment is esophagectomy
  - • Evaluate for retained foreign body

- ■ Treatment
  - • Give antibiotics immediately
  - • Surgery is indicated in all cases; if <24 hours, perform closure and drainage; if >24 hours, resect perforation, cervical esophagostomy, close distal esophagus, drain mediastinum, and jejunostomy
  - • Prognosis: survival rate is 90% when surgery is accomplished in <24 hours; survival drops to about 50% when treatment is delayed

- ■ Pearl
  Resect the esophagus if perforation has been present for >24 hours or if associated with underlying esophageal pathology.

Reference

Younes Z, Johnson DA: The spectrum of spontaneous and iatrogenic esophageal injury: Perforations, Mallory-Weiss tears, and hematomas. J Clin Gastroenterol 1999;29:306.

Esophageal Spasm, Diffuse

- **Essentials of Diagnosis**
  - Characterized by nonperistaltic esophageal contractions, often with chest pain
  - Symptoms and signs include chest pain, which is intermittent and varies from slight discomfort to severe spasmodic pain that simulates the pain of coronary artery disease; dysphagia for liquids and solids
  - Fluoroscopic studies show segmental spasms, areas of narrowing; manometry demonstrates repetitive, nonperistaltic (simultaneous) contractions after swallowing; provocative testing during manometry is positive if the anticholinesterase edrophonium, which causes strong esophageal contractions, elicits pain similar to the spontaneous symptom

- **Differential Diagnosis**
  - Heart disease, particularly coronary ischemia
  - Mediastinal masses
  - Benign and malignant esophageal tumors
  - Scleroderma

- **Treatment**
  - Surgery indications: esophageal myotomy for symptoms refractory to medical therapy; esophagectomy for persistent symptoms after myotomy
  - Esophageal dilation is ineffective
  - Medications: hydralazine, calcium channel blockers, long-acting nitrates, anticholinergic agents
  - Prognosis: esophageal myotomy is successful in 90% of cases; postoperative relief is associated with reduced intraluminal pressure

- **Pearl**

Always evaluate for underlying esophageal disease.

Reference

Ellis FH Jr: Long esophagomyotomy for diffuse esophageal spasm and related disorders: An historical overview. Dis Esophagus 1998;11:210.

Esophageal Sphincter Dysfunction, Upper

- **Essentials of Diagnosis**
  - Most often occurs in patients >60 years; may occur as an isolated abnormality or in association with Zenker diverticulum
  - Symptoms and signs include cervical dysphagia, more pronounced for solids than for liquids; chronic cough from minor aspirations of saliva and ingested food
  - Upper GI contrast radiography nearly always shows a prominent cricopharyngeal bar; endoscopy shows an extrinsic constriction; manometry often reveals imperfect coordination of relaxation of the cricopharyngeal sphincter

- **Differential Diagnosis**
  - Esophageal neoplasms
  - Reflux from lower esophageal sphincter incompetence

- **Treatment**
  - Myotomy of the cricopharyngeus and upper 3–4 cm of the esophageal musculature, made in the midline posteriorly
  - Surgery is indicated for all confirmed cases of upper esophageal sphincter dysfunction
  - Prognosis: relief of symptoms is usually complete and permanent after myotomy

- **Pearl**

Upper sphincter dysfunction and pharyngoesophageal (Zenker) diverticulum often coexist.

Reference

Owen W: ABC of the upper gastrointestinal tract. Dysphagia. BMJ 2001;323:850.

Esophageal Tumors, Benign

- **Essentials of Diagnosis**
  - May arise in any layer: mucosa, submucosa, muscularis propria
  - Mucosa: squamous papilloma is small, solitary, and sessile; fibrovascular polyps are pedunculated
  - Submucosa: lipoma, fibroma, hemangioma
  - Muscularis propria: leiomyoma is most common
  - Cysts: most are congenital foregut cysts
  - Symptoms and signs: often asymptomatic or cause mild dysphagia, pressure in neck or thorax, gastroesophageal reflux, chest pain, cough, dyspnea, regurgitation, upper GI bleeding
  - Barium swallow reveals a smooth, often spherical mass that causes extrinsic narrowing of the esophageal lumen; esophagoscopy is needed because leiomyomas arise from the deeper muscularis propria, and endoscopic biopsy often does not penetrate deeply enough to reach the tumor; endoscopic ultrasound identifies the layer from which tumor arises

- **Differential Diagnosis**
  - Leiomyomas and cysts can be distinguished from cancerous growths by their classic radiographic appearance
  - Intraluminal papillomas, granular cell tumors, and other benign tumors may be indistinguishable radiographically from early carcinoma, so their nature must be confirmed histologically

- **Treatment**
  - Most small, benign esophageal tumors can be removed endoscopically
  - Surgery is indicated for all symptomatic lesions or if unable to exclude carcinoma
  - Prognosis: low rate of recurrence and excellent prognosis after excision of benign esophageal tumors

- **Pearl**

Always rule out carcinoma, which is more common than the benign lesions.

Reference

Takada N et al: Utility of endoscopic ultrasonography in assessing the indications for endoscopic surgery of submucosal esophageal tumors. Surg Endosc 1999;13:228.

Esophagitis, Corrosive

- **Essentials of Diagnosis**
  - Strong alkali produces "liquefaction necrosis," which involves dissolution of proteins and collagen, saponification of fats, dehydration of tissues, thrombosis of blood vessels, and severe, deep penetrating injuries
  - Strong acid produces "coagulation necrosis," involving eschar formation, which tends to shield deeper tissues from injury
  - Liquid caustics usually produce more extensive esophageal injury than solids
  - Symptoms and signs include inflammatory edema of lips, mouth, tongue, and oropharynx; pain on attempted swallowing; chest pain; dysphagia; copious drooling; fever, shock, and peritoneal signs with esophageal perforation; possibly complete esophageal obstruction due to edema, inflammation, and mucosal sloughing
  - Esophagoscopy: scope should be inserted far enough to gauge the degree of burn but not beyond the proximal extent of injury
  - Esophageal burns can be classified by endoscopic appearance: grade I, superficial mucosal injury; grade II, partial-thickness injury; grade III, transmural injury with periesophageal or perigastric extension

- **Differential Diagnosis**
  - Rule out respiratory distress or severe pharyngeal injury with airway compromise necessitating intubation or tracheostomy; simultaneous gastric injury

- **Treatment**
  - Fluid resuscitation and airway protection
  - Surgery: laparotomy with resection of necrosis, cervical esophagostomy, oversewing of distal segment, feeding jejunostomy
  - Surgery is indicated for perforation; grade III injury; severe grade II injury; shock, peritonitis, worsening symptoms
  - Medications: do not attempt dilution or induce emesis; give antibiotics, H_2-receptor blockers
  - Prognosis: grade III, 20% mortality; with early endoscopy and aggressive treatment, mortality for less severe injury is low

- **Pearl**

Airway protection and suicide precautions must be considered.

Reference

de Jong AL et al: Corrosive esophagitis in children: A 30-year review. Int J Pediatr Otorhinolaryngol 2001;57:203.

Gastroesophageal Reflux Disease & Hiatal Hernia

- ■ Essentials of Diagnosis
  - • The principal barrier to reflux is the lower esophageal sphincter; competence is a function of sphincter pressure, sphincter length, and the length exposed to intra-abdominal pressure; bile acids may also play a role in esophagitis, especially in patients with previous gastric surgery
  - • Symptoms and signs include retrosternal and epigastric burning pain that occurs after eating and while sleeping or lying down and is relieved by drinking liquids, taking antacids, or standing or sitting up; regurgitation of bitter or sour-tasting fluid; pulmonary symptoms (wheezing, dyspnea) from aspiration
  - • Esophagoscopy and biopsy determine presence and degree of esophagitis and Barrett metaplasia; manometry shows decreased mean resting pressure in lower esophageal sphincter; pH monitoring reveals increased exposure of lower esophagus to acid, correlating with symptom onset

- ■ Differential Diagnosis
  - • Cholelithiasis
  - • Diverticulitis
  - • Peptic ulcer disease
  - • Achalasia
  - • Coronary artery disease

- ■ Treatment
  - • Asymptomatic hiatal hernia requires no treatment
  - • Fundoplication: intra-abdominal placement of gastroesophageal junction (GEJ) and buttressing of gastroesophageal sphincter
  - • Surgery is indicated for persistent or recurrent symptoms despite good medical therapy; development of strictures
  - • Medications: H_2-receptor blockers, proton pump inhibitors; recurrence is usual when drugs are discontinued
  - • Prognosis: 90% of patients experience a good result after surgery; 80–85% of cases of esophagitis heal after treatment with a proton pump inhibitor

- ■ Pearl

New-onset bronchospasm in an adult may be due to gastroesophageal reflux and minor, repeated pulmonary aspirations.

Reference

Watson DI et al: The changing face of treatment for hiatus hernia and gastroesophageal reflux. Gut 1999;45:791.

Mallory-Weiss Tear

- Essentials of Diagnosis
  - Responsible for about 10% of cases of acute upper GI hemorrhage; lesion is a 1- to 4-cm longitudinal tear in the gastric mucosa near the GEJ; about 75% of lesions are confined to the stomach, 20% straddle the GEJ, and 5% are entirely within the distal esophagus
  - Symptoms and signs: the patient first vomits food and gastric contents, followed by forceful retching and then bloody vomitus; epigastric pain; epigastric tenderness
  - Upper GI endoscopy shows gastric or distal esophageal mucosal tear with bleeding

- Differential Diagnosis
  - Rule out Boerhaave syndrome: actual rupture of the distal esophagus produced by vomiting
  - Other causes of upper GI hemorrhage

- Treatment
  - Bleeding can sometimes be controlled by endoscopic therapy; occasionally requires operative repair by gastrotomy and oversewing of tears
  - Surgery is indicated for persistent or recurrent bleeding after endoscopic treatment
  - Medications: H_2-receptor blockers, proton pump inhibitors to decrease risk of repeat bleeding
  - Prognosis: postoperative recurrence is rare

- Pearl

Always beware that another area in the upper GI tract can be the source of bleeding, despite demonstrated Mallory-Weiss tears.

Reference

Kortas DY: Mallory-Weiss tear: Predisposing factors and predictors of a complicated course. Am J Gastroenterol 2001;96:2863.

Paraesophageal Hiatal Hernia

- **Essentials of Diagnosis**
  - Acquired diaphragmatic defect containing variable amounts of stomach with or without other abdominal viscera; type II: rolling; upper dislocation of fundus of the stomach alongside a normally positioned intra-abdominal GEJ; type III: mixed; upper displacement of the fundus and GEJ; type IV: hernia contains other abdominal viscera
  - Symptoms and signs: often asymptomatic or causes pain or pressure in the lower chest after eating, vomiting, early satiety, hematemesis, dyspnea and pain on inspiration, decreased breath sounds in left chest, bowel sounds in left chest
  - Laboratory studies show anemia in 30% of patients
  - Chest film shows gastric air-fluid level behind cardiac shadow; upper GI contrast radiography demonstrates cephalad displacement of the stomach; endoscopy on retroversion shows orifice of the herniated portion of stomach adjacent to the GEJ (type II) or pouch with gastric rugal folds above the diaphragm with GEJ entering side of pouch (type III)

- **Differential Diagnosis**
  - Gastric volvulus
  - Strangulated viscera
  - Gastric necrosis

- **Treatment**
  - Surgery: herniated viscera are returned to the abdomen and enlarged hiatus is closed snugly around the GEJ; fundoplication may be performed to anchor the stomach or prevent reflux
  - Surgery is indicated because complications are frequent even in the absence of symptoms
  - Prognosis: excellent

- **Pearl**

Gastric ulcer often occurs at the area overriding the edge of the diaphragmatic defect, leading to chronic blood loss.

Reference

Luketich JD et al: Laparoscopic repair of giant paraesophageal hernia: 100 consecutive cases. Ann Surg 2000;232:608.

Pharyngoesophageal (Zenker) Diverticulum

- **Essentials of Diagnosis**
  - Diverticula are acquired lesions resulting from protrusion of mucosa and submucosa through a defect in the musculature due to high pressures generated during swallowing (pulsion type, most common) or from outward pulling of the esophagus from inflamed peribronchial mediastinal lymph nodes (traction type)
  - Symptoms and signs include dysphagia, related to size of the diverticulum; regurgitation of undigested food into the mouth, especially when patient is recumbent
  - Fluoroscopic examination shows a smoothly rounded, blind pouch; esophagoscopy is hazardous because the instrument may enter the ostium of the diverticulum and lead to perforation

- **Differential Diagnosis**
  - Malignant lesions
  - Achalasia of the cricopharyngeus muscle
  - Cervical esophageal webs (may accompany diverticula)

- **Treatment**
  - Surgery: excision of diverticulum and division of cricopharyngeal muscle
  - Other options: diverticulopexy; oropharyngeally placed ligating and dividing stapler
  - Surgery is indicated in all cases
  - Prevention: patient may manually massage the neck after eating to empty the sac
  - Prognosis: excellent

- **Pearl**

Zenker diverticulum may be associated with upper esophageal sphincter dysfunction.

Reference

Feeley MA et al: Zenker's diverticulum: Analysis of surgical complications from diverticulectomy and cricopharyngeal myotomy. Laryngoscope 1999;109:858.

Stomach & Duodenum

Duodenal Diverticula

- ■ Essentials of Diagnosis
  - Duodenal pulsion diverticula are acquired outpouchings of the mucosa and submucosa; found in 20% of autopsies and 5–10% of upper gastrointestinal (GI) series; 90% are on medial aspect of duodenum; most are solitary and within 2.5 cm of the ampulla of Vater
  - Symptoms are uncommon; patients may have chronic postprandial abdominal pain or dyspepsia; may present with symptoms from complications of diverticulum: hemorrhage, perforation, pancreatitis, biliary obstruction
  - Diverticulum is visualized on upper GI contrast radiographic studies or upper GI endoscopy

- ■ Differential Diagnosis
  - Other causes of upper GI perforation, bleeding, acute pancreatitis, or biliary obstruction

- ■ Treatment
  - Only 1% of cases found by x-ray warrant surgery
  - Operation includes excision and 2-layer closure
  - Endoscopic sphincterotomy or stent placement may be preferable to treat biliary obstruction
  - Surgery is indicated for all complications; severe persistent postprandial abdominal pain or dyspepsia
  - Prognosis: good with excellent surgical treatment of complications

- ■ Pearl

Most duodenal diverticula are asymptomatic and require no treatment.

Reference

Lobo DN et al: Periampullary diverticula and pancreaticobiliary disease. Br J Surg 1999;86:588.

Duodenal Tumors, Benign

- **Essentials of Diagnosis**
  - Adenomas are sessile or pedunculated; may be associated with familial adenomatous polyposis; types are tubular, villous, Brunner gland
  - Tubular: low malignant potential
  - Villous: high malignant risk; 30% of those >3 cm have malignant focus; often periampullary
  - Brunner gland: hyperplasia of exocrine glands
  - Gastrointestinal stromal tumor (GIST): difficult to distinguish benign from malignant on histologic studies
  - Hamartomas: associated with Peutz-Jeghers syndrome
  - Lipomas: no malignant potential
  - Symptoms and signs include gastric outlet obstruction, biliary obstruction and jaundice, upper GI bleeding
  - Duodenal tumor evident on upper GI endoscopy or contrast radiography

- **Differential Diagnosis**
  - Rule out malignant duodenal tumors or focus of malignancy within a largely benign lesion

- **Treatment**
  - Endoscopic removal if feasible
  - Surgery is indicated for failure of endoscopic removal or malignancy; pancreaticoduodenectomy usually indicated
  - Medications: imatinib mesylate for GIST
  - Prognosis: if benign, most tumors cured by complete removal; may recur after incomplete resection

- **Pearl**

About 50% of duodenal villous adenomas that are benign on endoscopic biopsy have focus of malignancy at resection.

Reference

Blanchard DK et al: Tumors of the small intestine. World J Surg 2000;24:421.

Duodenal Tumors, Malignant

■ Essentials of Diagnosis

- Adenocarcinoma: 67% periampullary; risk factors are Crohn disease, ulcerative colitis, polyposis syndromes, villous adenomas, hereditary nonpolyposis colon cancer
- Also include lymphoma; GIST (10–30% malignant)
- Symptoms and signs include abdominal pain, GI or biliary obstruction, GI bleeding (hematochezia or melena), weight loss; lymphoma: fever, night sweats, palpable abdominal mass
- Endoscopy and biopsy are usually diagnostic

■ Differential Diagnosis

- Rule out benign duodenal tumors

■ Treatment

- Pancreaticoduodenectomy is necessary for complete resection of most proximal duodenal malignancies
- Surgery is indicated for localized disease; resect all adenocarcinomas and GIST
- Medications: imatinib mesylate for GIST
- Prognosis: after curative resection, overall 5-year survival rate is 30%; for adenocarcinoma, 5-year survival for stage I is 80%; stage III, 10–15%

■ Pearl

About 50% of duodenal villous adenomas that are benign on endoscopic biopsy have focus of malignancy at resection.

References

Bakaeen FG et al: What prognostic factors are important in duodenal adenocarcinoma? Arch Surg 2000;135:635.

National Comprehensive Cancer Network: Practice Guidelines. http://www.nccn.org

Duodenal Ulcer

- ■ **Essentials of Diagnosis**
  - *Helicobacter pylori* infection is principal cause, making the duodenum more vulnerable to acid and pepsin; ulcer is most common in young and middle-aged patients (20–45 years); prevalence of duodenal ulcer reflects prevalence of *H pylori* infection; most patients infected with *H pylori* do not develop ulcer disease
  - Symptoms and signs include epigastric pain temporarily relieved by food, milk, or antacids; nausea, vomiting, and bleeding if ulcer perforates posterior duodenal wall; localized epigastric tenderness may be present on physical examination; many patients have few, vague abdominal symptoms
  - Laboratory findings: serum antibodies for *H pylori;* antral biopsy showing *H pylori* infection (histology, urease)
  - Imaging: esophagogastroduodenoscopy shows duodenal ulceration; radiographic upper GI contrast study shows ulcer niche, duodenal deformity, and distortion of duodenal bulb

- ■ **Differential Diagnosis**
  - Rule out Zollinger-Ellison syndrome (gastrinoma) in patients with severe or refractory duodenal ulcer

- ■ **Treatment**
  - Goals are to reduce acid secretion and eradicate *H pylori* infection
  - Surgery consists of parietal cell or truncal vagotomy with pyloroplasty; antrectomy and vagotomy
  - Surgery is indicated for intractable ulcer, failure of medical treatment, bleeding, perforation, duodenal obstruction
  - Medications: H_2-receptor blockers or proton pump inhibitors, antacids, treatment of *H pylori* infection
  - Prognosis: 80% heal within 6 weeks when treated with H_2-receptor blockers; 80% recurrence within 1 year if *H pylori* not eradicated
  - Prevention: avoid *H pylori* infection

- ■ **Pearl**

Operative treatment is rarely required for uncomplicated duodenal ulcer.

Reference

Jamieson GG: Current indications for surgery in peptic ulcer disease. World J Surg 2000;24:256.

Gastric Adenocarcinoma

■ **Essentials of Diagnosis**

- *H pylori* infection increases the risk of gastric cancer by 3.6- to 18-fold
- Morphologic types: ulcerating (15%), polypoid (25%), superficial spreading (15%), linitis plastica (10%), advanced (35%)
- Symptoms and signs include postprandial abdominal heaviness; early anorexia, with weight loss of about 6 kg; vomiting, often with blood, if pyloric obstruction occurs; epigastric mass in 25%; hepatomegaly in 10%; stool positive for occult blood in 50% but melena in a few
- Signs of distant spread: metastases to the neck (Virchow node) or umbilicus (Sister Mary Joseph node), metastases anterior to rectum detectable on rectal examination (Blumer shelf), metastases to ovaries (Krukenberg tumors)
- Laboratory findings: carcinoembryonic antigen is elevated in 65%; higher levels indicate extensive spread of tumor
- Endoscopy usually identifies gastric carcinomas

■ **Differential Diagnosis**

- Benign gastric ulcer, benign gastric tumors
- GIST, lymphoma

■ **Treatment**

- Surgery: resect tumor, adjacent margin of stomach (6 cm proximally) and duodenum, regional lymph nodes (no radical lymphadenectomy), and portions of adjacent organs if involved
- Curative resection is indicated if no metastases and reasonable operative risk; palliative resection if stomach is still movable and life expectancy is estimated at >1–2 months
- Medications: adjuvant chemotherapy after curative surgery not helpful; for advanced disease, chemotherapy ~20% response
- Prognosis: 5-year survival rates are 12% overall, 90% for early gastric cancer, 70% for stage I, 30% for stage II, 10% for stage III, 0% for stage IV

■ **Pearl**

Classic signs of distant spread are Virchow node, Sister Mary Joseph node, Blumer shelf, and Krukenberg tumor.

References

De Vivo R et al: Gastric cancer and *Helicobacter pylori:* A combined analysis of 12 case control studies nested within prospective cohorts. Gut 2001;49:347.
National Comprehensive Cancer Network: Practice Guidelines. http://www.nccn.org

Gastric Bezoar

- ■ Essentials of Diagnosis
    - Trichobezoar: composed of hair; usually found in young girls who pick at and swallow their hair
    - Phytobezoar: consists of agglomerated vegetable fibers, orange segments, or other fruits with a large amount of cellulose
    - Large semisolid bezoars of *Candida albicans* are rare in post-gastrectomy patients
    - Symptoms and signs include upper GI bleeding from gastric ulcer caused by pressure from mass, gastric perforation, abdominal pain
    - Upper GI endoscopy detects the bezoar and usually identifies its contents

- ■ Differential Diagnosis
    - Other causes of GI bleeding
    - Other causes of perforation

- ■ Treatment
    - Nearly all gastric bezoars can be dispersed by endoscopy
    - Surgery is indicated for inability to extract bezoar endoscopically, gastric bleeding, perforation
    - Prognosis: ulceration and bleeding are associated with 20% mortality

- ■ Pearl

Nearly all bezoars can be resolved endoscopically.

Reference

Lee J: Bezoars and foreign bodies of the stomach. Gastrointest Endosc Clin North Am 1996;6:605.

Gastric Lymphoma

- ■ Essentials of Diagnosis
  - Gastric lymphoma: second most common primary cancer of the stomach (2% of cases); most common site of extranodal lymphoma; associated with chronic *H pylori* infection; tumor usually bulky at presentation
  - Gastric pseudolymphoma: mass of lymphoid tissue in gastric wall often associated with an overlying mucosal ulcer
  - Symptoms and signs include epigastric pain and weight loss, nausea and vomiting, occult GI hemorrhage, palpable epigastric mass in 50%; pseudolymphoma presents similarly with pain and weight loss
  - Gastroscopy with biopsy and brush cytology provides the correct diagnosis preoperatively in about 75% of cases; computed tomography (CT) scan and bone marrow biopsy for preoperative staging

- ■ Differential Diagnosis
  - Gastric adenocarcinoma
  - Benign gastric ulcer
  - GIST

- ■ Treatment
  - Lymphoma: surgical resection and staging followed by total abdominal radiotherapy for localized disease; systemic chemotherapy for systemic disease
  - Pseudolymphoma: resection; no additional therapy
  - Splenectomy is indicated only if spleen is directly invaded
  - Medications: adjuvant radiation and chemotherapy for stage II and higher; eradication of *H pylori* for low-grade mucosa-associated lymphoid tissue tumor
  - Prognosis: 5-year disease-free survival is 50%; correlates with stage, grade, and extent of penetration of gastric wall; 60% of recurrences are extra-abdominal
  - Prevention: eradicate *H pylori*

- ■ Pearl

Always evaluate for systemic disease.

References

Kolve ME et al: Primary gastric non-Hodgkin's lymphoma: Requirement for diagnosis and staging. Recent Results Cancer Res 2000;156:63.

National Comprehensive Cancer Network: Practice Guidelines. http://www.nccn.org

Gastric Ulcer

■ **Essentials of Diagnosis**

- 85–90% of patients are infected with *H pylori*
- Morphology: type I ulcers (50%): located within 2 cm of incisura angularis; gastric acid output is normal or low; type II ulcers (20%): ulceration of both gastric body and duodenum; increased acid secretion; type III ulcers (20%): prepyloric location; increased acid secretion; type IV ulcers (5–10%): located high on lesser curvature at or near gastroesophageal junction; gastric acid output is normal or low; type V ulcers (<5%): due to nonsteroidal anti-inflammatory drug (NSAID) use
- Types I, IV, and V gastric ulcers are defects in mucosal protection; types II and III are associated with acid hypersecretion and behave like duodenal ulcers
- Symptoms and signs include epigastric pain, vomiting, anorexia, aggravation of pain by eating, occasional epigastric tenderness
- Workup: evaluate for *H pylori* infection
- Radiography or endoscopy shows gastric ulceration

■ **Differential Diagnosis**

- Ulcerated malignancy
- Zollinger-Ellison syndrome if disease is severe, refractory, or associated with more distal ulceration

■ **Treatment**

- Medications: treatment of *H pylori,* antacids, H_2-receptor blockers, proton pump inhibitors
- Surgery is rarely indicated except for complications or lack of healing (to rule out malignancy)
- Prognosis: excellent
- Prevention: treat *H pylori;* avoid NSAIDs

■ **Pearl**

Types I, IV, and V gastric ulcers are defects in mucosal protection; types II and III are associated with acid hypersecretion and behave like duodenal ulcers.

Reference

Calam J, Baron JH: ABC of the upper gastrointestinal tract: Pathophysiology of duodenal and gastric ulcer and gastric cancer. BMJ 2001;323:980.

Gastric Volvulus

- **Essentials of Diagnosis**
  - Rotation of the stomach about its longitudinal axis (organoaxial volvulus) or a line drawn from the mid lesser to the mid greater curvature (mesenteroaxial volvulus); organoaxial volvulus is more common and often associated with paraesophageal hiatal hernia
  - Symptoms and signs: acute volvulus causes severe abdominal pain, vomiting followed by retching and then inability to vomit, epigastric distention, inability to pass a nasogastric tube; chronic volvulus may be asymptomatic or cause crampy, intermittent abdominal pain
  - Upper GI contrast radiography demonstrates obstruction at the point of the volvulus

- **Differential Diagnosis**
  - Rule out other causes of upper GI obstruction

- **Treatment**
  - Immediate laparotomy for acute obstruction; if associated with paraesophageal hiatal hernia, should be treated by repair of hernia and anterior gastropexy
  - Surgery is indicated in all cases of gastric volvulus
  - Prognosis: good outcome if diagnosed and treated promptly, but mortality rate is high if gastric ischemia and necrosis develop

- **Pearl**

Acute gastric obstruction from volvulus is a surgical emergency.

Reference

Schaefer DC et al: Gastric volvulus: An old disease process with some new twists. Gastroenterologist 1997;5:41.

Gastrinoma (Zollinger-Ellison Syndrome)

- ■ Essentials of Diagnosis
  - • About 33% of cases associated with multiple endocrine neoplasia type 1
  - • Symptoms and signs mainly due to peptic ulcer disease from acid hypersecretion; ulcer symptoms are often refractory to antacids or H_2-blocking agents; some patients have severe diarrhea from large amounts of acid in duodenum, which can destroy pancreatic lipase, produce steatorrhea, damage small bowel mucosa, and overload intestine with gastric and pancreatic secretions
  - • Laboratory findings: hypergastrinemia (>500 pg/mL) with acid hypersecretion (H+ >15 mEq/h); gastrin >5000 pg/mL or α-chains of human chorionic gonadotropin in serum usually indicate metastasis; secretin provocative test for borderline gastrin values (200–500 pg/mL): a rise in gastrin level >150 pg/mL within 15 minutes is diagnostic
  - • CT or magnetic resonance imaging often detects pancreatic tumors; somatostatin-receptor scintigraphy is sensitive for gastrinoma primary and metastatic sites

- ■ Differential Diagnosis
  - • Gastric outlet obstruction, retained antrum, and antral cell hyperplasia (hypergastrinemia and gastric acid hypersecretion)
  - • Pernicious anemia, atrophic gastritis, gastric ulcer, and postvagotomy state (hypergastrinemia without acid in stomach)

- ■ Treatment
  - • Suppress gastric acid output before any other therapy
  - • Surgical resection is indicated in all patients with apparently localized disease
  - • Medications: H_2-receptor blockers, proton pump inhibitors; maintain gastric H+ output <5 mEq in hour before next dose
  - • Prognosis: 70% of patients have biochemical cure after resection; 30% of patients disease-free after 5 years; patients with multiple endocrine neoplasia type 1 rarely cured

- ■ Pearl

Gastrinoma diagnosis must document simultaneous hypergastrinemia and acid in the stomach.

References

National Comprehensive Cancer Network: Practice Guidelines. http://www.nccn.org
Norton JA et al: Surgery to cure the Zollinger-Ellison syndrome. N Engl J Med 1999;341:635.

Ménétrièr Disease

- ■ Essentials of Diagnosis
  - Giant hypertrophy of gastric rugae with excess loss of protein from thickened mucosa into the gut, with resulting hypoproteinemia; increased risk of adenocarcinoma of stomach in adults; associated with *H pylori* infection
  - Symptoms and signs include diarrhea, indigestion, anorexia, weight loss, skin rash, edema from hypoproteinemia, symptomatic anemia
  - On upper GI contrast studies, hypertrophic rugae create enormous filling defects, frequently misinterpreted as carcinoma; also apparent on upper GI endoscopy

- ■ Differential Diagnosis
  - Rule out adenocarcinoma

- ■ Treatment
  - Goal is to reduce protein loss
  - Surgery is total gastrectomy
  - Surgery is rarely indicated for severe intractable hypoproteinemia, anemia, or inability to exclude cancer
  - Prognosis: despite medical support and *H pylori* eradication, gastric abnormalities and hypoproteinemia may persist

- ■ Pearl

Most patients can be managed nonoperatively.

Reference

Madsen LG et al: Ménétrièr's disease and *Helicobacter pylori*: Normalization of gastrointestinal protein loss after eradication therapy. Dig Dis Sci 1999;44:2307.

Peptic Ulcer Hemorrhage

- **Essentials of Diagnosis**
  - Most common cause of massive upper GI hemorrhage; chronic gastric and duodenal ulcers have about the same tendency to bleed, but more severe bleeding with gastric ulcers; bleeding duodenal ulcers usually located on posterior surface of duodenal bulb with erosion into gastroduodenal artery; gastric ulcers rebleed 3 times more commonly than duodenal ulcers
  - Symptoms and signs include epigastric pain, abdominal tenderness; acute hemorrhage causes hematemesis or hematochezia, hypotension or shock; chronic hemorrhage causes weakness, anemia, fecal occult blood
  - Upper GI endoscopy shows bleeding ulcer, visible vessel, ulcer with adherent clot

- **Differential Diagnosis**
  - Esophageal varices
  - Gastritis
  - Mallory-Weiss syndrome
  - Gastric cancer

- **Treatment**
  - Replace blood loss with crystalloid and blood products; nasogastric lavage; endoscopy for localization and possible treatment
  - Surgery is indicated for massive hemorrhage with shock, ongoing transfusion requirements (>6 U packed red blood cells), recurrent hemorrhage
  - Surgery: excise ulcer (gastric) or oversew vessel (duodenal); consider vagotomy to acutely decrease mucosal blood flow
  - Medications: H_2-receptor blockers, proton pump inhibitors (may reduce risk of rebleeding)
  - Prognosis: 75% managed by endoscopy alone; surgery required in <10% of cases; 15% mortality from massive hemorrhage

- **Pearl**

Delay of operation beyond 6 U of blood loss is associated with increased operative morbidity.

Reference

Rockall TA: Management and outcome of patients undergoing surgery after acute upper gastrointestinal haemorrhage. Steering Group for the National Audit of Acute Upper Gastrointestinal Haemorrhage. J R Soc Med 1998;91:518.

Peptic Ulcer Perforation

- **Essentials of Diagnosis**
  - Perforation complicates peptic ulcer about half as often as hemorrhage; most perforated ulcers are located anteriorly
  - Symptoms and signs: usually sudden, severe upper abdominal pain; patient is severely distressed, lying quietly with knees drawn up and breathing shallowly to minimize abdominal motion; fever develops within 12–24 hours; rebound tenderness and abdominal rigidity; reduced or absent bowel sounds; free air in abdomen with abdominal distention and diffuse tympany
  - Laboratory studies show mild leukocytosis of about 12,000/μL in early stages, followed by rise to 20,000/μL within 12–24 hours; infection with *H pylori*
  - Abdominal x-ray reveals free intraperitoneal air in 85% of patients

- **Differential Diagnosis**
  - Simultaneous onset of pain and free air without trauma or endoscopy usually indicates perforated peptic ulcer
  - Rule out acute pancreatitis and acute cholecystitis, free perforation of colonic diverticulitis, acute appendicitis (rare)

- **Treatment**
  - Surgery: all free perforations should be repaired by secure closure with omentum (Graham patch closure); addition of parietal cell vagotomy or truncal vagotomy and pyloroplasty versus treatment of *H pylori* is controversial
  - Surgery is indicated in nearly all cases; rare patient with sealed perforation may be managed without operation
  - Medications: treatment of *H pylori* infection; H_2-receptor blockers, proton pump inhibitors; antibiotics (cefazolin, cefoxitin)
  - Prognosis: 15% mortality, mostly from delay in treatment, advanced age, and comorbid diseases

- **Pearl**

Simultaneous onset of pain and free air without trauma or endoscopy usually indicates perforated peptic ulcer.

Reference

Svanes C: Trends in perforated peptic ulcer: Incidence, etiology, treatment, and prognosis. World J Surg 2000;24:277.

Polyps, Gastric

- **Essentials of Diagnosis**
  - Hyperplastic polyps (>80%): represent overgrowth of normal epithelium, with no relationship to gastric cancer
  - Adenomatous polyps: 30% contain a focus of adenocarcinoma; about 10% of benign adenomatous polyps undergo malignant change during prolonged follow-up
  - Symptoms and signs: most are asymptomatic or cause vague epigastric discomfort, dyspepsia, occult GI bleeding, gastric outlet obstruction with nausea and vomiting if polyp is located in distal stomach
  - Upper GI endoscopy reveals gastric polyp

- **Differential Diagnosis**
  - Rule out gastric cancer

- **Treatment**
  - Endoscopic removal is successful in most cases; laparotomy or laparoscopy if endoscopy is unsuccessful
  - Resection if cancer is found in polyp
  - Gastrectomy may be required for multiple polyps
  - Prognosis: recurrent polyps are uncommon

- **Pearl**

Removal is indicated to fully evaluate for malignancy.

Reference

Abraham SC et al: Hyperplastic polyps of the stomach: Associations with histologic patterns of gastritis and gastric atrophy. Am J Surg Pathol 2001;25:500.

Pyloric Obstruction

- ■ Essentials of Diagnosis
  - Duodenal ulcer is a more common cause of obstruction than gastric ulcer; usually a history of symptomatic peptic ulcer disease
  - Symptoms and signs include increasing ulcer pain with anorexia, vomiting of undigested food, and failure to gain relief from antacids; absence of bile pigment in vomitus reflects level of duodenal obstruction; weight loss, dehydration, and malnutrition may be marked; peristalsis of distended stomach may be visible; upper abdominal distention and tenderness usually apparent; tetany with advanced alkalosis; possible infection with *H pylori*
  - Contrast radiographic upper GI series shows retention of contrast proximal to the obstruction; gastroscopy reveals luminal narrowing; indicated to evaluate for obstructing neoplasm

- ■ Differential Diagnosis
  - Obstruction due to peptic ulcer must be differentiated from malignant tumor of antrum, duodenum, or pancreas

- ■ Treatment
  - Replace fluid and electrolytes; place nasogastric tube for decompression
  - If conservative management fails, perform drainage and consider truncal or parietal cell vagotomy
  - Surgery is indicated for failure of obstruction to resolve completely within 5–7 days; recurrent obstruction of any degree
  - Medications: H_2-receptor blockers, proton pump inhibitors; treatment of *H pylori* infection; total parenteral nutrition for malnutrition
  - Prognosis: about 67% of patients with acute obstruction fail to improve with medical therapy and require operation

- ■ Pearl

Operation is usually required to resolve obstruction.

Reference

Jamieson GG: Current status of indications for surgery in peptic ulcer disease. World J Surg 2000;24:256.

Stress Ulcer

- ■ Essentials of Diagnosis
  - Causes include shock, sepsis, burns (Curling ulcers), tumors or trauma of central nervous system (Cushing ulcers); clinically apparent ulcers develop in about 20% of susceptible patients; most stress ulcers develop in the stomach, 30% in the duodenum, and sometimes both
  - Symptoms and signs: hemorrhage is nearly always initial manifestation; clinically evident bleeding usually 3–5 days after injury; massive bleeding generally 4–5 days later; pain is rare; physical examination is not contributory except for gross or occult fecal blood or signs of shock
  - Gastroduodenal endoscopy shows shallow, discrete ulcers in stomach, duodenum, or both

- ■ Differential Diagnosis
  - Rule out other causes of GI hemorrhage

- ■ Treatment
  - Gastric lavage; endoscopic treatment of bleeding ulcers; infusion of vasopressin into left gastric artery through percutaneous catheter may be useful; suture of bleeding points, vagotomy, and antrectomy or pyloroplasty; rarely, total gastrectomy is necessary
  - Medications: H_2-receptor blockers may decrease rebleeding; blood or crystalloid infusion as indicated
  - Prognosis: overall mortality determined largely by underlying disease
  - Prevention: far preferable to treatment; H_2-receptor blockers or sucralfate prophylactically for critically ill patients

- ■ Pearl

Prevention is far preferable to treatment.

Reference

Felig DM, Carafa CJ: Stress ulcers of the stomach. Gastrointest Endosc 2000;51:596.

16

Pancreas

Annular Pancreas

- **Essentials of Diagnosis**
  - Ring of pancreatic tissue from head of the pancreas surrounding the descending duodenum, leading to obstruction; presents in infancy or adulthood
  - Symptoms and signs include upper gastrointestinal (GI) obstruction, vomiting, upper GI bleeding, epigastric pain
  - Upper GI contrast radiography shows narrowing of duodenum where it is encircled by the pancreatic head, with proximal dilation; endoscopic retrograde cholangiopancreatography (ERCP) shows pancreatic duct in head of pancreas encircling the duodenum

- **Differential Diagnosis**
  - Duodenal tumors
  - Pancreatic head masses
  - Duodenal atresia (infants)

- **Treatment**
  - Bypass obstructed segment by duodenojejunostomy; do not resect obstructing pancreas because of high risk of pancreatic fistula
  - Surgery is indicated in all cases in children and all symptomatic cases in adults; if obstruction is discovered incidentally in an asymptomatic adult, no treatment is needed
  - Prognosis: excellent after surgical bypass of obstruction

- **Pearl**

  If obstruction is discovered incidentally in an asymptomatic adult, no treatment is needed.

Reference

McCollum MO et al: Annular pancreas and duodenal stenosis. J Pediatr Surg 2002;37:1776.

Glucagonoma

- ■ Essentials of Diagnosis
  - Arises from cells in the pancreatic islets; most tumors are solitary and large (>4 cm), located in body or tail of the pancreas; about 25% are benign and confined to the pancreas
  - Symptoms and signs include migratory necrolytic dermatitis, usually involving the legs and perineum; weight loss; stomatitis; thrombophlebitis
  - Laboratory tests reveal elevated serum glucagon level (>100 pg/mL), hypoaminoacidemia, anemia, hyperglycemia
  - Computed tomography (CT) scan or magnetic resonance imaging (MRI) demonstrates the tumor and sites of metastases

- ■ Differential Diagnosis
  - Diagnosis is suspected from the distinctive skin lesion
  - Also suspect glucagonoma in any patient with new onset of diabetes after age 60 years
  - Rule out other causes of dermatitis; other pancreatic islet cell tumors

- ■ Treatment
  - Surgical resection of primary tumor; depends on location: distal subtotal pancreatectomy and splenectomy for tail and body; pancreaticoduodenectomy (Whipple) for head of pancreas
  - Medications: total parenteral nutrition, somatostatin analogues (octreotide) for symptomatic palliation, streptozocin and dacarbazine for unresectable lesions, anticoagulation for thrombophlebitis
  - Prognosis: good with complete resection of tumor; palliation can be achieved with resection and debulking of metastatic disease

- ■ Pearl

The rash is effectively treated with octreotide.

References

Chastain MA: The glucagonoma syndrome: A review of its features and discussion of new perspectives. Am J Med Sci 2001;321:306.

National Comprehensive Cancer Network: Practice Guidelines. http://www.nccn.org

Insulinoma

- **Essentials of Diagnosis**
  - 75% are solitary and benign; 10% are malignant; metastases are usually evident at diagnosis; patients with multiple endocrine neoplasia type 1 may have insulinomas as one of several tumors
  - Symptoms and signs include palpitations, sweating, tremulousness, weight gain, bizarre behavior, memory lapse, unconsciousness
  - Laboratory tests show fasting hypoglycemia with inappropriately high levels of insulin; ratio of plasma insulin to glucose is >0.3, with serum glucose <40 mg/dL diagnostic; proinsulin levels >40% suggest a malignant islet cell tumor; elevated C-peptide levels exclude self-administration of insulin; absent urine sulfonylurea excludes oral hypoglycemic agents
  - Endoscopic ultrasound of the pancreas identifies 80–95% of tumors preoperatively; intraoperative ultrasound can identify pancreatic tumor in nearly all cases and is the gold standard

- **Differential Diagnosis**
  - Rule out non-islet cell tumors associated with hypoglycemia (hemangiopericytoma, fibrosarcoma, leiomyosarcoma, hepatoma, adrenocortical carcinoma)
  - Exclude surreptitious self-administration of insulin or oral hypoglycemic agents

- **Treatment**
  - Enucleation of tumor if accessible and away from the duct, or resection as part of a partial pancreatectomy if deemed less morbid
  - Surgery is indicated in all patients with resectable lesions
  - Medications: diazoxide or octreotide to suppress insulin release; streptozocin is the best chemotherapeutic agent
  - Prognosis: patients with benign sporadic insulinomas are cured with resection; 60% of patients with malignant disease live up to 2 more years

- **Pearl**

Whipple triad: hypoglycemia with symptoms of neuroglycopenia relieved by glucose administration.

Reference

Grant CS: Surgical aspects of hyperinsulinemic hypoglycemia. Endocrinol Metab Clin North Am 1999;28:533.

Islet Cell Tumors, Nonfunctioning

- ■ Essentials of Diagnosis
  - Account for 30–50% of pancreatic endocrine tumors; most are large, malignant, and located in head of the pancreas; metastases are present at diagnosis in 80% of patients
  - Symptoms and signs include abdominal and back pain, weight loss, jaundice, nausea and vomiting, palpable abdominal mass
  - Laboratory tests can show elevated serum chromogranin A, pancreatic polypeptide, and human chorionic gonadotropin
  - CT scan demonstrates a mass, typically hypervascular; also useful for detecting metastases; octreotide scintigraphy shows sites of disease and somatostatin receptor content of tumor

- ■ Differential Diagnosis
  - Functional islet cell tumors
  - Adenocarcinoma of head of the pancreas
  - Chronic pancreatitis

- ■ Treatment
  - Resection of primary tumor: head, pancreaticoduodenectomy; body and tail, distal pancreatectomy; debulking of metastases
  - Surgery is indicated for all completely resectable disease
  - Medications: streptozocin and doxorubicin for unresectable tumor
  - Prognosis: 5-year disease-free survival rate is 15%

- ■ Pearl

Chromogranin A may be a useful tumor marker for follow-up.

Reference

Bartsch DK et al: Management of nonfunctioning islet cell carcinomas. World J Surg 2000;24:1418.

Pancreatic Abscess

- **Essentials of Diagnosis**
  - Abscess complicates about 5% of cases of acute pancreatitis and carries high mortality rate; abscess forms after secondary bacterial contamination of necrotic pancreatic debris and hemorrhagic exudates
  - Symptoms and signs include epigastric pain, palpable tender mass, fever, jaundice (if biliary obstruction occurs from inflammation)
  - Laboratory tests indicate leukocytosis, elevated bilirubin; aspirated fluid should be tested with Gram stain and culture
  - CT scan reveals fluid collection in affected area of pancreas; gas in the fluid collection suggests infection
  - Workup: perform percutaneous CT-guided aspiration to obtain specimen for Gram stain and culture

- **Differential Diagnosis**
  - Rule out uninfected pancreatic necrosis, which may not require surgical treatment

- **Treatment**
  - Percutaneous drainage is inadequate; surgical drainage and debridement of necrotic pancreatic debris followed by external drainage are required
  - Surgery is indicated in all cases of infected pancreatic abscess; sterile pancreatic necrosis as an indication for operation is controversial
  - Medications: broad-spectrum antibiotics
  - Prognosis: mortality rate is 20%, usually because of severe abscess, incomplete surgical drainage, and delayed diagnosis

- **Pearl**

Infected pancreatic necrosis requires surgical debridement for complete drainage.

Reference

Tsiotos GG, Sarr MG: Management of fluid collections and necrosis in acute pancreatitis. Curr Gastroenterol Rep 1999;1:139.

Pancreatic Adenocarcinoma

- ■ Essentials of Diagnosis
  - Third leading cancer in men aged 35–54 years; incidence and mortality are roughly equal, underscoring the abysmal prognosis
  - Symptoms and signs include weight loss; abdominal pain; back pain (worse prognosis); nausea and vomiting; migratory thrombophlebitis; palpable epigastric mass; obstructive jaundice, often with pruritus or cholangitis; palpable, nontender gallbladder in right upper quadrant (Courvoisier sign); sudden onset of diabetes mellitus in 25% of patients
  - Laboratory examination shows elevated serum levels of CA 19-9 (sensitivity too low to use as a screening tool)
  - CT scan shows pancreatic mass, dilated pancreatic duct or bile duct; ERCP demonstrates stenosis or obstruction of pancreatic duct or bile duct ("double-duct sign"); CT findings suggesting unresectable tumor: local tumor extension, contiguous organ invasion, distant metastases, involvement of the superior mesenteric or portal vessels, ascites

- ■ Differential Diagnosis
  - Chronic pancreatitis
  - Other periampullary neoplasms: carcinoma of the ampulla of Vater, distal common bile duct, or duodenum
  - Retroperitoneal lymphoma; retroperitoneal sarcoma

- ■ Treatment
  - For curable lesions of the head, pancreaticoduodenectomy (Whipple); laparoscopy may be useful to identify unresectable disease without morbidity of laparotomy
  - Surgery is indicated for any lesion suspicious for pancreatic cancer
  - Medications: radiation therapy with chemotherapy (gemcitabine): neoadjuvant, adjuvant, palliative; celiac plexus block for pain
  - Prognosis: mean survival after palliative therapy is 7 months; after potentially curative resection, 18 months; with clear margins, 20% of patients live >5 years; overall 5-year survival is <3%

- ■ Pearl

The surgeon's annual pancreatectomy volume predicts mortality from the Whipple procedure.

References

Farnell MB et al: The Mayo Clinic approach to the surgical treatment of adeno-carcinoma of the pancreas. Surg Clin North Am 2001;81:611.

National Comprehensive Cancer Network: Practice Guidelines. http://www.nccn.org

Pancreatic Ascites & Pancreatic Pleural Effusion

- **Essentials of Diagnosis**
  - Accumulated pancreatic fluid in the abdomen or chest, originating from a pancreatic fistula, without peritonitis or severe pain; most often due to chronic leakage of a pseudocyst; rarely due to disruption of a pancreatic duct (trauma)
  - Symptoms and signs include marked weight loss, abdominal distention (ascites), respiratory difficulty (effusion)
  - Laboratory findings: the fluid ranges in appearance from straw-colored to blood-tinged; contains elevated protein (>2.9 g/dL) and amylase (usually >3000 IU/dL)
  - Small leaks not detected by ERCP may be imaged by CT scan performed immediately after ERCP while contrast medium is still in pancreatic duct

- **Differential Diagnosis**
  - Ascites from underlying hepatic disease
  - Pleural effusion from underlying pulmonary disease

- **Treatment**
  - Fluid drainage and chest tube (effusion); limited oral intake, total parenteral nutrition, somatostatin
  - Surgery consists of internal drainage; endoscopic stenting of pancreatic duct may be successful
  - Surgery is indicated if no improvement after 2–3 weeks of medical treatment or recurrence after removal of chest tube
  - Prognosis: excellent with therapy; death rate is low in patients treated before debilitation becomes severe

- **Pearl**

Treatment depends on decreasing fistula output (limiting pancreatic fluid production and decreasing resistance to flow through ampulla) to allow scarring and closure of fistula tract.

Reference

Kaman L et al: Internal pancreatic fistulas with pancreatic ascites and pancreatic pleural effusions: Recognition and management. Aust N Z J Surg 2001;71:221.

Pancreatic Insufficiency

- ■ Essentials of Diagnosis
  - • Usually due to pancreatectomy or pancreatic disease, particularly chronic pancreatitis
  - • Symptoms and signs include fat malabsorption and steatorrhea; diarrhea may be present; weight loss may occur from caloric malnutrition; signs and symptoms of underlying disease (chronic pancreatitis)
  - • Laboratory examination of stool specimen for fat globules is specific and relatively sensitive for fat malabsorption

- ■ Differential Diagnosis
  - • Dumping syndrome
  - • Infectious diarrhea

- ■ Treatment
  - • Diet plan for 3000–6000 kcal/d, emphasizing carbohydrate ($\geq$400 g) and protein (100–150 g); dietary restriction of fat is important to control diarrhea
  - • No surgical intervention is indicated
  - • Medications: pancrelipase replacement; H_2-receptor blockers to retard gastric acid destruction of lipase; medium-chain triglycerides
  - • Prognosis: symptoms often improve with pancreatic enzyme replacement

- ■ Pearl

A trial of pancrelipase and time is often helpful.

Reference

DiMagno EP: Gastric acid suppression and treatment of severe exocrine pancreatic insufficiency. Best Pract Res Clin Gastroenterol 2001;15:477.

Pancreatic Neoplasms, Cystic

- Essentials of Diagnosis
  - Four major types: mucinous cystic neoplasm, serous cystic neoplasm, intraductal papillary mucinous neoplasm, solid pseudopapillary tumor
  - Mucinous cystic neoplasm (1–2% of pancreatic tumors): 2:1 female predominance; most in body or tail of pancreas; usually diagnosed in fourth or fifth decade; high malignant potential for mucinous cystadenocarcinoma
  - Serous cystic neoplasm (1–2% of pancreatic tumors): 2:1 female predominance; usually diagnosed in seventh decade; rarely malignant
  - Intraductal papillary mucinous neoplasm (<1% of pancreatic tumors): commonly in women <25 years old; most in tail of pancreas; metastases in 10–15% at presentation; seldom invasive
  - Symptoms and signs include epigastric mass, abdominal pain, jaundice if tumor obstructs biliary tract; intraductal papillary mucinous neoplasm may cause acute pancreatitis
  - CT scan: mucinous cystic neoplasm: unilocular or multilocular cyst; serous cystic neoplasm: honeycomb pattern of microcysts; intraductal papillary mucinous neoplasm: cyst communicates with often dilated pancreatic duct; solid pseudopapillary tumor: sharply circumscribed with thick pericystic fibrous capsule

- Differential Diagnosis
  - Rule out pancreatic pseudocyst if associated with acute or chronic pancreatitis

- Treatment
  - Pancreatic resection if possible
  - Prognosis: mucinous cystic neoplasm: 70% survival at 5 years; serous cystic neoplasm: resection is curative; intraductal papillary mucinous neoplasm: survival >60% at 5 years; solid pseudopapillary tumor: 95% are cured with resection

- Pearl

Intraductal papillary mucinous neoplasm often includes microscopic infiltration of adjacent tissue; resection must be complete.

References

National Comprehensive Cancer Network: Practice Guidelines. http://www.nccn.org
Sarr MG et al: Cystic neoplasms of the pancreas: Benign to malignant epithelial neoplasms. Surg Clin North Am 2001;81:497.

Pancreatic Pseudocyst

- **Essentials of Diagnosis**
  - Encapsulated collection of pancreatic secretions; causes include acute pancreatitis, chronic ductal obstruction (chronic pancreatitis), or acute ductal disruption (trauma)
  - Walls of pseudocyst are formed by inflammatory fibrosis of peritoneal, mesenteric, and serosal membranes, which limit spread of pancreatic juice as lesion develops
  - Symptoms and signs: abdominal pain is most common; fever; weight loss; jaundice from obstruction of intrapancreatic segment of bile duct; palpable, tender mass in the epigastrium
  - CT scan is diagnostic study of choice, showing size and shape of the cyst and relationship to other viscera; ERCP should be performed if obstruction or disruption of pancreatic duct, as these findings require endoscopic or surgical treatment

- **Differential Diagnosis**
  - Pancreatic abscess, acute pancreatic phlegmon, pancreatic adenocarcinoma
  - Neoplastic cysts account for about 5% of cystic pancreatic masses; may be indistinguishable preoperatively from pseudocyst; if operative drainage is performed, biopsy cyst wall to exclude neoplasia

- **Treatment**
  - Asymptomatic cysts may be observed; 40% will resolve within 8–12 weeks
  - Drainage options: internal (cystgastrostomy or jejunostomy), external, percutaneous (if infected)
  - Surgery is indicated for all symptomatic pseudocysts, cysts >5 cm that have not resolved 8–12 weeks after acute pancreatitis, infected pseudocysts (external surgical or percutaneous drainage)
  - Monitor expectant management with interval CT or ultrasound to document resolution; if no resolution or if symptoms develop, drainage is indicated
  - Prognosis: recurrence rate is about 10%; higher after external drainage; surgery is usually uncomplicated and definitive

- **Pearl**

The vast majority of acute pseudocysts resolve spontaneously.

Reference

Cooperman AM: Surgical treatment of pancreatic pseudocysts. Surg Clin North Am 2001;81:411.

Pancreatitis, Acute

- ■ Essentials of Diagnosis
  - Nonbacterial inflammatory disease of activation, interstitial liberation, and enzymatic autodigestion of pancreas
  - Biliary: 40% of cases; if untreated, high risk of additional acute attacks; alcoholic: 40% of cases; other causes: hypercalcemia, hyperlipidemia, familial, iatrogenic, drug-induced, obstructive, idiopathic
  - Symptoms and signs include severe epigastric pain radiating to the back; nausea and vomiting; tachycardia and postural hypotension; normal or slightly elevated temperature; distention and generalized or epigastric tenderness; decreased or absent bowel sounds; abdominal mass due to pancreatic phlegmon, pseudocyst, or abscess; ecchymosis in flank (Grey Turner sign) or periumbilical area (Cullen sign) from retroperitoneal dissection of blood
  - Laboratory tests show mild elevation of serum bilirubin, greater with choledocholithiasis; elevated serum amylase; elevated serum lipase; decreased serum calcium; base deficit or hypoxemia
  - CT scan useful for severe illness or if no improvement after 48–72 hours; may demonstrate phlegmon, necrosis, pseudocyst, or abscess; abdominal ultrasound may show gallstones, dilated common bile duct, or choledocholithiasis (biliary pancreatitis)

- ■ Differential Diagnosis
  - Necrotizing pancreatitis, infected necrotizing pancreatitis, pancreatic abscess
  - Other causes: acute cholecystitis, penetrating or perforated duodenal ulcer, high small bowel obstruction, acute appendicitis, mesenteric infarction, chronic hyperamylasemia

- ■ Treatment
  - Limit enteral intake, perform nasogastric suction, replace fluids, correct electrolytes, treat underlying cause
  - For biliary pancreatitis, perform cholecystectomy after resolution but before hospital discharge
  - Prognosis: acute pancreatitis has 10% mortality; necrotizing pancreatitis, 50% mortality

- ■ Pearl

Respiratory insufficiency and hypocalcemia indicate a poor prognosis.

Reference

Dervenis C, Bassi C: Evidence-based assessment of severity and management of acute pancreatitis. Br J Surg 2000;87:257.

Pancreatitis, Chronic

- ■ Essentials of Diagnosis
  - • May be familial (familial pancreatitis) or due to chronic partial obstruction of pancreatic duct, which is either congenital (pancreas divisum) or due to injury (trauma) or inflammation (alcoholic chronic pancreatitis)
  - • Pathologic changes in gland include destruction of parenchyma, fibrosis, dedifferentiation of acini, calculi, ductal dilation
  - • Symptoms and signs include severe pain, typically deep in the upper abdomen and radiating to the back; pain varies from day to day; malabsorption and steatorrhea
  - • Serum amylase may be elevated in acute exacerbations
  - • CT scan shows pancreatic calcification, stones in and dilation of pancreatic duct, and dilated bile duct if obstructed; ERCP shows pancreatic ductal stones, irregularity with dilation and stenoses, and occasionally ductal occlusion; bile duct dilation due to smooth compression of intrapancreatic duct by cicatrix

- ■ Differential Diagnosis
  - • Pancreatic pseudocyst
  - • Pancreatic adenocarcinoma

- ■ Treatment
  - • Surgery for pancreatic drainage: longitudinal pancreaticoje-junostomy if duct is dilated (Puestow); pancreaticoduodenectomy if duct not dilated and disease mainly in head; total pancreatectomy for failure of other procedures
  - • Surgery is indicated for chronic, intractable pain; relief of pain with endoscopic stenting of pancreatic duct may predict patients who will benefit from operation
  - • Medications: celiac plexus block; pancreatic enzymes
  - • Prognosis: pain relief with longitudinal pancreaticojejunostomy and pancreaticoduodenectomy successful in 80% of patients; celiac plexus block in <30% of patients

- ■ Pearl

Many patients with chronic pain from pancreatitis develop narcotic addiction, which requires management in addition to the pancreatitis.

Reference

Apte MV et al: Chronic pancreatitis: Complications and management. J Clin Gastroenterol 1999;29:225.

Somatostatinoma

- **Essentials of Diagnosis**
  - Accounts for 1–2% of pancreatic islet cell tumors; results from secretion of somatostatin by an islet cell tumor of the pancreas; most tumors are malignant and accompanied by hepatic, regional lymph node, and bone metastases; mean age at presentation is 50 years; men and women are affected equally
  - Symptoms and signs include diarrhea, steatorrhea, weight loss
  - Laboratory testing shows increased plasma somatostatin
  - Lesion is usually large and readily demonstrated by CT scan; abdominal ultrasound may show gallbladder dilation with cholelithiasis

- **Differential Diagnosis**
  - Other islet cell tumors of the pancreas
  - Other causes of diarrhea and malabsorption

- **Treatment**
  - Surgical enucleation; pancreaticoduodenectomy for lesions in head of the pancreas; distal subtotal pancreatectomy for lesions in tail
  - Surgery is indicated for all resectable lesions; debulking of hepatic metastases for relief of symptoms
  - Medications: chemotherapy with streptozocin, dacarbazine, or doxorubicin for unresectable tumors
  - Prognosis: when disease is localized, resection cures about 50% of patients

- **Pearl**

Octreotide is ineffective for treating the somatostatinoma hormonal syndrome.

References

National Comprehensive Cancer Network: Practice Guidelines. http://www.nccn.org

Soga J, Yakuwa Y: Somatostatinoma/inhibitory syndrome: A statistical evaluation of 173 reported cases as compared to other pancreatic endocrinomas. J Exp Clin Cancer Res 1999;18:13.

VIPoma

- ■ Essentials of Diagnosis
  - Non-beta islet cell tumor of the pancreas that secretes vasoactive intestinal peptide (VIP); VIPomas cause the WDHH syndrome (watery diarrhea, hypokalemia, hypochlorhydria); approximately 80% of the tumors are solitary, located in body or tail of pancreas; about 50% are malignant, and 75% of those have metastasized by the time of exploration
  - Symptoms and signs include profuse watery diarrhea, extreme weakness
  - Laboratory studies show elevated fasting VIP levels (>190 pg/mL), hypokalemia, severe metabolic acidosis from loss of HCO_3 in the stool
  - CT scan or MRI is the best initial test for localizing tumor and metastases; somatostatin receptor scintigraphy also useful
  - Workup: document secretory diarrhea (stool volume averages ~5 L/d during acute episodes; not resolved by stopping oral intake), serum VIP level, CT scan or MRI

- ■ Differential Diagnosis
  - Other causes of diarrhea: infections, short bowel syndrome, medications, pancreatic insufficiency
  - Other tumors: gastrinoma, carcinoid tumor, medullary thyroid cancer

- ■ Treatment
  - Resection of entire tumor; palliative debulking of metastases
  - Surgery is indicated in all cases if technically feasible
  - Medications: octreotide is extremely effective at palliating the hormonal syndrome; long-acting somatostatin analogues (every 4 weeks) decrease VIP levels, control diarrhea, and may reduce tumor size
  - Prognosis: 1-year survival is 40% in patients with unresectable tumor

- ■ Pearl

Always control tumor syndrome before operation.

References

National Comprehensive Cancer Network: Practice Guidelines. http://www.nccn.org

Soga J, Yakuwa Y: Vipoma/diarrheogenic syndrome: A statistical evaluation of 241 reported cases. J Exp Clin Cancer Res 1998;17:389.

17

Spleen

Felty Syndrome

- ■ Essentials of Diagnosis
  - • Affects patients with seropositive nodular rheumatoid arthritis; recurrent infections are due to decreased and dysfunctional neutrophils coated with immunoglobulin G (IgG)
  - • Symptoms and signs include recurring infections, splenomegaly, chronic leg ulcers
  - • Laboratory studies show decreased neutrophil count, increased granulopoiesis in bone marrow, high levels of IgG on surface of neutrophils

- ■ Differential Diagnosis
  - • Other causes of neutropenia: aplastic anemia, pure white cell aplasia, drugs (sulfonamides, procainamide, penicillin, cyclosporines, cimetidine, phenytoin, chlorpropamide)
  - • Sepsis
  - • Immune mediated

- ■ Treatment
  - • Splenectomy removes source of antibody-mediated neutrophil destruction
  - • Surgery is indicated for patients with recurrent bacterial infections and evidence of IgG on surface of neutrophils
  - • Prognosis: neutropenia improves in 60–70% after splenectomy; recurrence is possible; splenectomy beneficial even if no postoperative increase in neutrophil count

- ■ Pearl

Always evaluate for other causes of neutropenia.

Reference

Logue GL et al: Failure of splenectomy in Felty's syndrome. N Engl J Med 1981;304:580.

Hemolytic Anemia, Acquired

- **Essentials of Diagnosis**
  - Autoimmune disorder that is either idiopathic (40–50%) or secondary to drug exposure, connective tissue diseases, or lymphoproliferative disorders; most common after age 50 years; occurs twice as often in women as in men
  - Symptoms and signs include fatigue, mild jaundice, fever, splenomegaly
  - Laboratory examination demonstrates acute-onset normocytic normochromic anemia, reticulocytosis (>10%), erythroid hyperplasia of the marrow, elevation of serum indirect bilirubin, usually low or absent serum haptoglobin, positive direct Coombs test

- **Differential Diagnosis**
  - Hereditary hemolytic anemias
  - Thrombotic thrombocytopenic purpura
  - Disseminated intravascular coagulation
  - Infection

- **Treatment**
  - Drug-induced hemolytic anemia: terminate exposure to the agent
  - Splenectomy is indicated for patients with warm-antibody hemolysis who fail to respond to 4–6 weeks of high-dose corticosteroid therapy, relapse after corticosteroids are withdrawn, or have contraindications to corticosteroids
  - Medications: corticosteroids; intravenous immune globulin
  - Prognosis: 75% remission rate with medical treatment; 25% of remissions are permanent; relapses may occur after splenectomy

- **Pearl**

Most patients can be treated without splenectomy.

Reference

Beutler E et al: Hemolytic anemia. Semin Hematol 1999;36:38.

Hemolytic Anemias, Miscellaneous Hereditary

- ■ Essentials of Diagnosis
    - • Hereditary elliptocytosis: elliptical erythrocytes due to defects in cytoskeletal proteins, leading to change in shape, decreased plasticity, and shortened lifespan
    - • Hereditary nonspherocytic hemolytic anemia: due to inherited red cell defects that lead to oxidative hemolysis (pyruvate kinase deficiency and glucose 6-phosphate dehydrogenase deficiency)
    - • Thalassemia major and minor: structural defect in β-globin chain causes excess α-chains to precipitate and cells to pass poorly through spleen, leading to increased splenic destruction and target cells; heterozygotes usually have mild anemia (thalassemia minor); homozygotes have severe chronic anemia starting in infancy
    - • Symptoms and signs include abdominal pain, jaundice, splenomegaly
    - • Laboratory studies show anemia, increased serum bilirubin, decreased haptoglobin, increased reticulocyte count; hereditary elliptocytosis: elliptical red blood cells (RBCs) on peripheral smear; thalassemia: target cells, nucleated red cells, and hypochromic microcytic anemia on peripheral smear; persistence of fetal hemoglobin

- ■ Differential Diagnosis
    - • Other causes of hemolytic anemia: autoimmune hemolytic anemias, thrombotic thrombocytopenic purpura, disseminated intravascular coagulation
    - • Infection

- ■ Treatment
    - • Splenectomy may reduce transfusion requirements and abdominal pain of splenomegaly; if gallstones are present, then concurrent cholecystectomy
    - • Surgery is indicated in all cases
    - • Prognosis: transfusion requirements may be decreased and abdominal pain improved after splenectomy

- ■ Pearl

Always consider cholecystectomy if operation is planned.

References

Silveira P et al: Red blood cell abnormalities in hereditary elliptocytosis and their relevance to variable clinical expression. Am J Clin Pathol 1997;108:391.
Weatherall DJ: The thalassemias. BMJ 1997;314:1675.

Immune Thrombocytopenic Purpura

- ### Essentials of Diagnosis
  - Caused by a circulating antiplatelet IgG autoantibody; spleen is both the site of platelet destruction and source of autoantibody; disease is idiopathic or secondary to lymphoproliferative disorder, drugs or toxins, bacterial or viral infection (especially in children), systemic lupus erythematosus
  - Symptoms and signs include ecchymoses or showers of petechiae, bleeding gums, vaginal bleeding, gastrointestinal bleeding, hematuria
  - Laboratory findings: platelet count is low (<100,000/µL); bone marrow shows increased numbers of large megakaryocytes; bleeding time is prolonged; partial thromboplastin time, prothrombin time, and coagulation time are normal; iron deficiency anemia is a result of bleeding

- ### Differential Diagnosis
  - Other causes of nonimmunologic thrombocytopenia: leukemia, aplastic anemia, macroglobulinemia
  - Thrombocytopenia and purpura may be caused by ineffective thrombocytopoiesis (pernicious anemia), nonimmune platelet destruction (septicemia, disseminated intravascular coagulation, hypersplenism)

- ### Treatment
  - Patients with mild or no symptoms need no specific therapy
  - Corticosteroids initially; splenectomy is effective; no platelet transfusions unless active bleeding
  - Surgery is indicated for failure to respond to corticosteroids, relapse after initial remission on corticosteroids, corticosteroid dependence
  - Prognosis: splenectomy achieves sustained remission in 60–90% of patients; corticosteroid response is 70–80%; sustained remissions in 20% of adults

- ### Pearl
  Intraoperative bleeding is uncommon even with low platelet count; delay platelet transfusion until splenic vessels are divided.

Reference

George JN et al: Idiopathic thrombocytopenic purpura: Diagnosis and management. Am J Med Sci 1998;316:87.

Postsplenectomy Sepsis

- ■ Essentials of Diagnosis
  - • Persons are susceptible to fulminant bacteria after splenectomy because of decreased clearance of encapsulated bacteria from the blood, decreased levels of IgM, decreased opsonic activity; risk of fatal sepsis is higher when splenectomy performed for hematologic disorders rather than trauma, probably because of autotransplantation; *Streptococcus pneumoniae, Haemophilus influenzae,* and meningococci are most common pathogens
  - • Symptoms and signs include mild, nonspecific symptoms followed by high fever and shock from sepsis, which may rapidly lead to death

- ■ Differential Diagnosis
  - • Underlying cause of sepsis must be diagnosed and treated; the course of sepsis is more fulminant than with spleen intact

- ■ Treatment
  - • Therapy is directed to the underlying infection
  - • To avoid the situation, defer splenectomy until age 6 years unless the hematologic problem is especially severe; avoid splenectomy or perform partial splenectomy or splenic repair for ruptured spleen to maintain adequate splenic function
  - • Prevention: preoperative vaccination against pneumococci and *H influenzae* type b; prophylactic ampicillin (age <6 years)
  - • Prognosis: survival is improved with early recognition and aggressive treatment of infection

- ■ Pearl
  Early recognition of the infection can provide time for therapy; patient and family education regarding the risk is critical.

Reference

Brigden ML et al: Prevention and management of overwhelming postsplenectomy infection—an update. Crit Care Med 1999;27:836.

Spherocytosis

- ■ **Essentials of Diagnosis**
  - • The most common congenital hemolytic anemia, affecting 1 in 5000 persons; caused by deficiency of spectrin and ankyrin, erythrocyte membrane proteins that maintain cellular osmotic stability and prevent splenic destruction
  - • Symptoms and signs include mild to moderate anemia, jaundice, easy fatigability, discomfort in left upper quadrant, splenomegaly
  - • Laboratory tests show decreased RBC count and hemoglobin; negative Coombs test; spherocytes on Wright-stained smear; increased reticulocyte count (5–20%); elevated indirect serum bilirubin and stool urobilinogen; decreased or absent serum haptoglobin; increased osmotic fragility, best demonstrated by cryohemolysis test

- ■ **Differential Diagnosis**
  - • Spherocytes in large numbers may occur in autoimmune hemolytic anemias, with increased osmotic fragility and autohemolysis
  - • Spherocytes are also present in hemoglobin C disease, in some alcoholics, and in some severe burns

- ■ **Treatment**
  - • Splenectomy, with cholecystectomy if associated cholelithiasis
  - • Surgery is indicated for all patients >6 years, even if asymptomatic
  - • Prognosis: splenectomy cures anemia and jaundice; the membrane abnormality and increased osmotic fragility persist, but RBC lifespan is almost normal

- ■ **Pearl**

Delay splenectomy to age 6 years to limit the risk of postsplenectomy sepsis.

Reference

Marchetti M et al: Prophylactic splenectomy and cholecystectomy in mild hereditary spherocytosis: Analyzing the decision in different clinical scenarios. J Intern Med 1998;244:217.

Splenic Abscess

- ■ Essentials of Diagnosis
  - Causes include hematogenous seeding of the spleen with bacteria from remote septic focus (endocarditis, intra-abdominal infection), direct spread of infection from adjacent structures (pancreatic or perinephric abscess, diverticulitis, colon or gastric perforation), splenic trauma or infarction with secondarily infected hematoma or necrotic parenchyma
  - Laboratory culture shows *Staphylococcus* species, 20%; *Salmonella,* 15%; anaerobic bacteria, 15%; *Escherichia coli,* 10–15%; *Streptococcus* species, 10%; *Enterococcus* species, 5–10%
  - Computed tomography (CT) scan demonstrates fluid-filled lesion, possibly containing gas

- ■ Differential Diagnosis
  - Subphrenic abscess, perinephric abscess
  - Splenic tumor or cyst

- ■ Treatment
  - Broad-spectrum antibiotics
  - Splenectomy is essential for cure if sepsis is localized to the spleen; percutaneous drainage of large, solitary juxtacapsular abscess may be feasible
  - Prognosis: 85–95% of cases are treated successfully with splenectomy; 75% of selected cases are treated successfully with percutaneous drainage

- ■ Pearl

Evaluate for other sites of disseminated infection.

Reference

Phillips GS et al: Splenic abscess: Another look at an old disease. Arch Surg 1997;132:1331.

Splenic Cysts & Tumors

- **Essentials of Diagnosis**
  - Malignant primary tumors: non-Hodgkin lymphoma (NHL), angiosarcoma
  - Benign splenic tumors: hemangioma, lymphangioma, inflammatory pseudotumor
  - Splenic cysts: true parasitic cysts (5%), usually hydatid—*Echinococcus granulosus;* true nonparasitic cysts (15%), epidermoid is most common; pseudocysts (80%), post-trauma or infarction
  - Symptoms and signs: NHL: splenomegaly, constitutional symptoms; angiosarcoma, metastatic tumor, true cysts (parasitic or not), and pseudocysts: abdominal pain, palpable abdominal mass; inflammatory pseudotumor: fever, malaise, weight loss; hemangiomas and lymphangiomas: usually asymptomatic
  - CT scan shows splenic mass; NHL: splenomegaly with solitary mass (>5 cm) or multiple masses; angiosarcoma: solitary mass with central tumor necrosis; hemangioma: well-circumscribed nodules with enhancement, cystic changes, and calcifications; lymphangiomas: multiple cysts; pseudocysts: round, well-circumscribed unilocular cyst, may have a calcified rim

- **Differential Diagnosis**
  - Malignant splenic tumor or abscess

- **Treatment**
  - Splenectomy for all primary malignant tumors and parasitic cysts; partial or complete splenectomy for benign tumors and cysts if symptomatic, risk for rupture, or otherwise indicated
  - Surgery is indicated for abdominal pain, splenomegaly, hypersplenism with cytopenia; metastatic tumors if solitary; pseudocysts if symptoms or >10 cm
  - Prognosis: NHL: similar to other forms of NHL; angiosarcomas: poor; benign tumors and cysts: cured with splenectomy

- **Pearl**

Evaluate for other sites of systemic disease for infectious or malignant splenic lesions.

Reference

Du Plessis DG et al: Mucinous epithelial cysts of the spleen associated with pseudomyxoma peritonei. Histopathology 1999;52:333.

Splenic Neoplasms

- ■ Essentials of Diagnosis
  - • Chronic lymphocytic leukemia: neoplasm of B cells
  - • Hairy cell leukemia: low-grade lymphoproliferative disorder
  - • Idiopathic myelofibrosis: extensive bone marrow fibrosis and extramedullary hematopoiesis
  - • Mast cell disease: rare condition of mast cell infiltration of tissues
  - • Symptoms and signs: chronic lymphocytic leukemia: fatigue, splenomegaly, lymphadenopathy, bleeding; hairy cell leukemia: splenomegaly, infections, bleeding, fatigue; idiopathic myelofibrosis: weakness and fatigue, dyspnea, splenomegaly, abdominal fullness and pain, bleeding, infection; mast cell disease: splenomegaly, bleeding

- ■ Differential Diagnosis
  - • Other causes of hypersplenism and cytopenias: Waldenström macroglobulinemia, NHL, Hodgkin disease, chronic myelogenous leukemia

- ■ Treatment
  - • Splenectomy
  - • Surgery is indicated for splenomegaly with abdominal pain, hypersplenism with cytopenias, as adjunct to medical treatment, failure of medical treatment, portal hypertension (idiopathic myelofibrosis)
  - • Prognosis: splenectomy relieves symptoms of splenomegaly in most cases; cytopenias are corrected in 50–75% of cases; 80–95% of patients with hairy cell leukemia respond to medical therapy

- ■ Pearl

Morbidity is increased after any procedure in patients with idiopathic myelofibrosis.

Reference

Thiruvengadam R et al: Splenectomy in advanced chronic lymphocytic leukemia. Leukemia 1990;4:758.

Splenosis

- **Essentials of Diagnosis**
  - Solitary splenic implants have little clinical significance; usually an incidental finding at laparotomy for an unrelated problem; implants are capable of cell culling and some immunologic function
  - Symptoms and signs: asymptomatic, except in patients with spleen-dependent anemia (immune thrombocytopenic purpura)
  - Laboratory findings include absence of Howell-Jolly bodies: characteristic post-splenectomy RBC nuclear remnants that are typically removed by the spleen
  - CT scan shows implants as small peritoneal or mesenteric nodules

- **Differential Diagnosis**
  - Peritoneal nodules of metastatic carcinoma; accessory spleen
  - Histologically, splenosis differs from accessory spleen by the absence of elastic or smooth muscle fibers in the delicate capsule

- **Treatment**
  - No treatment is warranted for uncomplicated splenosis
  - Recurrent immune thrombocytopenic purpura may rarely require attempt at removal of implants
  - Prognosis: usually an incidental finding of little significance

- **Pearl**

Meticulous anatomic removal of the spleen without capsular or hilar disruption is important if leaving splenic implants would be deleterious.

Reference

Pisters PWT et al: Autologous splenic transplantation for splenic trauma. Ann Surg 1994;219:225.

Thrombotic Thrombocytopenia Purpura

- ■ Essentials of Diagnosis
  - Cause is unknown; believed to be an autoimmune response to endothelial cell antigen in small vessels
  - Symptoms and signs include fever, purpura, and ecchymosis; neurologic changes of headache, confusion, aphasia, lethargy, hemiparesis, seizures, and coma; hepatomegaly; splenomegaly; bleeding
  - Laboratory studies show thrombocytopenia, anemia, increased lactate dehydrogenase, reticulocytosis, increased bilirubin, decreased haptoglobin, negative Coombs test, fragmented RBCs on peripheral smear

- ■ Differential Diagnosis
  - Disseminated intravascular coagulation
  - Evans syndrome
  - Endocarditis, vasculitis
  - Immune thrombocytopenic purpura

- ■ Treatment
  - Plasmapheresis with plasma exchange, corticosteroids, antiplatelet agents
  - Splenectomy can be adjunct to medical treatment to reduce platelet and RBC losses
  - Surgery is indicated for medically refractory or recurrent disease
  - Medications: corticosteroids, antiplatelet drugs (aspirin and dipyridamole)
  - Prognosis: 65% remission with splenectomy alone; combined therapy achieves prolonged remission in most patients

- ■ Pearl

The anemia is often severe, and it may be aggravated by hemorrhage secondary to thrombocytopenia.

Reference

Rock GA: Management of thrombotic thrombocytopenic purpura. Br J Haematol 2000;109:496.

18

Small Intestine

Blind Loop Syndrome

- **Essentials of Diagnosis**
  - Intestinal stasis and bacterial overgrowth related to disruption of propulsive forces or other factors that limit bacterial growth; strictures, diverticula, fistulas, or poorly emptying segments of intestine cause stagnation and permit bacterial proliferation
  - Symptoms and signs include steatorrhea, diarrhea, malnutrition
  - Laboratory findings include megaloblastic anemia; impaired absorption of orally administered vitamin B_{12}; ^{14}C-D-xylose breath test: anaerobic bacteria in small bowel metabolize xylose, releasing $^{14}CO_2$, which is detected in the breath
  - Upper gastrointestinal (GI) contrast radiographic study or computed tomography (CT) scan may reveal blind intestinal loop, intestinal stricture, or fistula

- **Differential Diagnosis**
  - Short bowel syndrome
  - Small intestinal lymphoma
  - Pancreatic exocrine insufficiency
  - Inflammatory bowel disease

- **Treatment**
  - Surgery for underlying fistula, blind loop, diverticula, or other lesion; or broad-spectrum antibiotics and drugs to control diarrhea
  - Surgery is indicated for anatomic defects amenable to treatment: fistula, diverticulum, blind loop
  - Medications: antibiotics, antidiarrheal agents
  - Prognosis: good if anatomic defect is identified and corrected

- **Pearl**

Avoid the creation of blind loops during operation.

Reference

Rubesin SE et al: Small-bowel malabsorption: Clinical and radiologic perspectives. How we see it. Radiology 1992;184:297.

Crohn Disease

- ■ Essentials of Diagnosis
    - Chronic progressive granulomatous inflammatory disorder affecting any part of GI tract; distal ileum is most frequently involved, eventually becoming diseased in 75% of cases
    - Symptoms and signs include diarrhea, which contains no blood if small bowel alone is diseased; acute and recurrent abdominal pain; malaise; weight loss; malnutrition; fever; palpable abdominal mass; abdominal tenderness; anorectal lesions: chronic anal fissures, large ulcers, complex anal fistulas, or pararectal abscesses
    - Upper GI contrast radiography shows thickened bowel wall with stricture, longitudinal ulceration, deep transverse fissures, cobblestone formation; fistulas and abscesses may be detected

- ■ Differential Diagnosis
    - Ulcerative colitis
    - Appendicitis
    - Tuberculosis (TB)
    - Lymphoma
    - Carcinoma
    - Amebiasis
    - Ischemia
    - Eosinophilic gastroenteritis

- ■ Treatment
    - Surgery may manage complications in coordination with medical therapy and is palliative, not curative
    - Surgery is indicated for obstruction, perforation, internal or external fistula or abscess, growth failure in children
    - Medications: steroids, aminosalicylates, immunosuppressive agents, and metronidazole (perianal disease); infliximab
    - Prognosis: symptomatic recurrence rates after resection are 15–50% at 5 years, 35–80% at 10 years, 45–85% at 15 years

- ■ Pearl

The inflammation of Crohn disease does not respect anatomic borders, leading to abscesses and enteroenteral and enterocutaneous fistulas.

Reference

Ricart E et al: Infliximab for Crohn's disease in clinical practice at the Mayo Clinic: The first 100 patients. Am J Gastroenterol 2001;96:722.

Ileus

- ■ Essentials of Diagnosis
  - • Adynamic ileus is a functional obstruction due to dysmotility of the bowel; must differentiate ileus from mechanical bowel obstruction; dysfunction is due to a combination of neural, hormonal, and metabolic factors
  - • Symptoms and signs include abdominal tenderness, abdominal distention, hypoactive or absent bowel sounds, absence of flatus or passage of stool

- ■ Differential Diagnosis
  - • Mechanical causes of bowel obstruction

- ■ Treatment
  - • Treatment is conservative; no oral intake, nasogastric (NG) decompression, intravenous (IV) hydration; correct electrolyte abnormalities; discontinue or substitute for narcotic pain medications or psychotropic medications if possible
  - • Prognosis: time and correction of underlying causes should allow resolution of ileus
  - • Prevention: meticulous technique in operating room, minimal use of narcotics for analgesia, correction of electrolyte or metabolic imbalance, early recognition of septic complications

- ■ Pearl

Ileus is common and usually resolves with time.

Reference

Shelton AA et al: Small intestine. In Way LW, Doherty GM (editors): Current Surgical Diagnosis & Treatment, 11th ed. McGraw-Hill, 2003.

Intussusception, Adult

- **Essentials of Diagnosis**
  - Invagination of proximal intestine into adjacent distal bowel, resulting in luminal obstruction; a lead point is often identified in adults and must be sought in all patients
  - Symptoms and signs include clinical evidence of bowel obstruction: colicky abdominal pain, vomiting, hyperperistaltic bowel sounds
  - Barium enema may be both diagnostic and therapeutic: "coiled spring" sign; resolution of obstruction after contrast enema (often not possible in adults)
  - Workup: evaluate patient thoroughly to identify the anatomic lead point

- **Differential Diagnosis**
  - Neoplasm
  - Hernia
  - Adhesions
  - Diverticulitis
  - Appendicitis

- **Treatment**
  - Surgical reduction is usually required; IV hydration; NG decompression; IV broad-spectrum antibiotics; barium or air-contrast enema
  - At operation, reduce intussusception by pushing the lead point, avoiding pulling; if reduction cannot be done without creating serosal tears, perform resection and anastomosis in the absence of gross contamination
  - Prognosis: recurrence rates are 1–3% whether barium or operative reduction is performed; death can occur rarely if treatment of gangrenous bowel is delayed

- **Pearl**

Intussusception in adults usually has an anatomic abnormality as the lead point.

Reference

Shelton AA et al: Small intestine. In Way LW, Doherty GM (editors): Current Surgical Diagnosis & Treatment, 11th ed. McGraw-Hill, 2003.

Pneumatosis Intestinalis

■ Essentials of Diagnosis

- Gas-filled cysts in wall of intestine and mesentery; may be primary and idiopathic, an incidental finding, or secondary to chronic obstructive pulmonary disease, infectious gastroenteritis, or connective tissue disorders
- Causes of secondary pneumatosis intestinalis include inflammatory bowel disease, infectious gastroenteritis, corticosteroid therapy, connective tissue disorders, intestinal obstruction, diverticulitis, chronic obstructive pulmonary disease, acute leukemia, lymphoma, acquired immunodeficiency syndrome, organ transplantation
- Symptoms and signs include abdominal discomfort, diarrhea, excessive flatus, abdominal distention, abdominal tenderness
- Abdominal x-rays and CT scan show linear gas deposits in intestinal wall; if perforation is present, free air may be visualized

■ Differential Diagnosis

- Intestinal ischemia
- Strangulation obstruction

■ Treatment

- Primary and secondary pneumatosis: no specific treatment; oxygen administration may speed resolution
- Fulminant pneumatosis: bowel resection
- Surgery is indicated for intestinal necrosis, intestinal ischemia, strangulation obstruction
- Prognosis: primary and secondary have excellent outcome; fulminant has high mortality rate from intestinal necrosis

■ Pearl

Pneumatosis is usually a sign of significant primary bowel wall ischemia.

Reference

Hoover EL et al: Avoiding laparotomy in nonsurgical pneumoperitoneum. Am J Surg 1992;164:99.

Short Bowel Syndrome

- **Essentials of Diagnosis**
  - May develop after extensive resection of small intestine
  - When ≤3 m of small intestine remains, serious nutritional abnormalities develop
  - When ≤2 m remains, function is clinically impaired in most patients but with time, normal function may return
  - When ≤1 m remains, many patients require parenteral nutrition permanently
  - Because transport of bile salts, vitamin B_{12}, and cholesterol is localized to ileum, resection of this region is poorly tolerated; steatorrhea and diarrhea are more pronounced if ileocecal valve is removed
  - Symptoms and signs include diarrhea (>2 L/d of fluid and electrolyte losses)
  - Laboratory studies show hemoconcentration, metabolic acidosis, hypokalemia, hypocalcemia
  - GI contrast radiographic studies show decreased intestinal length and decreased transit time

- **Differential Diagnosis**
  - Blind loop syndrome
  - Small intestine lymphoma
  - Pancreatic exocrine insufficiency
  - Inflammatory bowel disease

- **Treatment**
  - Initially, limit enteral intake and give total parenteral nutrition; resume oral feedings when diarrhea subsides to <2.5 L/d while continuing IV nutrition
  - Prognosis: intestinal adaptation and oral intake can be achieved in most patients

- **Pearl**

Adaptation takes time; maintain adequate nutrition with parenteral support while intestine adjusts to limited enteral nutrition.

Reference

Chris Anderson-Hill D, Heimburger DC: Medical management of the difficult patient with short-bowel syndrome. Nutrition 1993;9:536.

Small Intestine Carcinoid

- ■ Essentials of Diagnosis
    - Arises from neuroendocrine cells throughout the gut and produces endocrine and vasoactive substances; hepatic metastases usually necessary to produce the carcinoid syndrome
    - Symptoms and signs: small tumors are usually asymptomatic; bowel obstruction is due to mesenteric desmoplastic reaction; abdominal pain, GI bleeding, intestinal ischemia, abdominal tenderness; carcinoid syndrome: cutaneous flushing, diarrhea, bronchoconstriction, right-sided cardiac valvular disease
    - Laboratory studies show elevated urinary levels of 5-hydroxyindoleacectic acid
    - CT scan shows mesenteric nodal or hepatic metastases, hypervascular lesions; somatostatin receptor scintigraphy demonstrates extent of disease and somatostatin receptors on tumor

- ■ Differential Diagnosis
    - Other neuroendocrine tumors
    - Benign and malignant small intestine tumors

- ■ Treatment
    - Surgery: all accessible carcinoid tumors should be resected for cure or palliation; localized hepatic metastases should be resected
    - Medications: octreotide and histamine antagonists for carcinoid syndrome
    - Prognosis: 70% overall 5-year survival rate; 14-year median survival from time of diagnosis; 8-year median survival from onset of carcinoid syndrome

- ■ Pearl

Octreotide effectively palliates carcinoid syndrome in nearly all patients.

References

National Comprehensive Cancer Network: Practice Guidelines. http://www.nccn.org
Søreide O et al: Surgical treatment as a principle in patients with advanced abdominal carcinoid tumors. Surgery 1992;111:48.

Small Intestine Diverticula

- ■ Essentials of Diagnosis
  - Acquired diverticula occur in 1.3% of the population; Meckel diverticulum is a congenital, true diverticulum that results from persistence of vitelline duct and occurs on antimesenteric border of ileum; Meckel rule of 2: occurs in males twice as often as females, occurs in 2% of population, becomes symptomatic in 2% of cases, occurs 2 feet proximal to the ileocecal valve, may extend over 2 inches in length, can cause 2 symptoms: bleeding and obstruction
  - Symptoms and signs: most are asymptomatic; symptoms may be due to obstruction, inflammation, bleeding, or bacterial overgrowth; abdominal pain; GI hemorrhage; diarrhea and malabsorption
  - CT scan may reveal diverticula and associated inflammation or obstruction; for Meckel diverticulum, [99]technetium-pertechnate scan can identify ectopic gastric mucosa in the diverticulum

- ■ Differential Diagnosis
  - Other causes of GI bleeding
  - Small bowel obstruction
  - Small bowel inflammation

- ■ Treatment
  - Asymptomatic diverticula require no treatment
  - Small bowel resection and anastomosis for complications
  - Prognosis: diverticula are treated completely by segmental small bowel resection

- ■ Pearl

Asymptomatic diverticula require no treatment.

Reference

Longo WE, Vernava AD: Clinical implications of jejunoileal diverticular disease. Dis Colon Rectum 1992;35:381.

Small Intestine Enteropathies, Noninfectious

- **Essentials of Diagnosis**
  - NSAID enteropathy: nonsteroidal anti-inflammatory drugs (NSAIDs) increase intestinal permeability, leading to mucosal inflammation; enteropathy with subclinical intestinal inflammation and occult blood loss develops in 70% of patients who have taken NSAIDs for >6 months
  - Radiation enteropathy: injury to blood vessels in bowel wall leads to endothelial proliferation and fibrosis that obliterate the vessel lumen, producing chronic intestinal ischemia; symptoms may appear as early as 1 month or as late as 30 years after completion of therapy
  - Symptoms and signs include nausea and vomiting; abdominal pain; GI bleeding; diarrhea, which may be bloody; abdominal tenderness
  - CT scan shows dilated bowel with bowel wall edema proximal to the obstruction; narrowed, stenotic bowel at the site of obstruction; free air suggests perforation

- **Differential Diagnosis**
  - Crohn disease
  - Ischemia
  - TB
  - Lymphoma
  - Primary or recurrent carcinoma

- **Treatment**
  - NSAID enteropathy: discontinue drug
  - Radiation enteropathy: no effective therapy; management is supportive for nutrition and bowel obstruction
  - Surgery is indicated for complications
  - Prognosis: good for NSAID enteropathy after medication is discontinued; symptoms of acute radiation enteropathy are usually minor and transient, but can be followed by chronic scarring

- **Pearl**

Operative treatment of radiation enteropathy is reserved for significant focal complications because the diffuse effects are not remediable.

Reference

Cross MJ, Frazee RC: Surgical treatment of radiation enteritis. Am Surg 1992;58:132.

Small Intestine Fistulas

- ■ Essentials of Diagnosis
  - May form spontaneously as a result of disease (Crohn disease), but >95% are surgical complications
  - Symptoms and signs include fever, abdominal pain before bowel movement, rapid weight loss, abdominal tenderness
  - Contrast medium administered orally, per rectum, or through fistula (fistulogram) delineates abnormal anatomy (including intrinsic bowel disease) and demonstrates location and number of fistulas, length and course of fistula tracts, associated abscess cavities, and distal obstruction; CT scan may identify associated abscesses and allow percutaneous drainage

- ■ Differential Diagnosis
  - Associated carcinoma
  - Inflammatory bowel disease
  - Anastomotic disruption
  - GI perforation, distal GI obstruction

- ■ Treatment
  - Replace fluids, electrolytes, and nutrients; protect skin from excoriation; drain abscess; avoid enteral intake; perform NG suction
  - Many fistulas will heal unless distal obstruction, cancer, foreign body, or underlying cause of Crohn disease, radiation or tuberculous enteritis
  - Surgery: resect fistulous segment, relieve associated obstruction, reestablish continuity by end-to-end anastomosis
  - Surgery is indicated for persistence >1 month; postpone operation until intra-abdominal inflammation has resolved, typically 2–3 months after most recent operation
  - Medications: H_2-receptor blockers, octreotide, total parenteral nutrition
  - Prognosis: with proper management, survival rates are 80–95%; uncontrolled sepsis is chief cause of death

- ■ Pearl

Healing is impaired by distal obstruction, cancer, foreign body, or underlying cause of Crohn disease or radiation or tuberculous enteritis.

Reference

Borison DI et al: Treatment of enterocutaneous and colocutaneous fistulas with early surgery or somatostatin analog. Dis Colon Rectum 1992;35:635.

Small Intestine Tumors, Benign

- **Essentials of Diagnosis**
  - Adenomas: tubular: low malignant potential, can cause obstruction or intussusception; villous: significant malignant potential, associated with inherited colonic polyposis syndromes; Brunner gland: no malignant potential
  - Stromal tumors: mesenchymal neoplasms, the most common symptomatic benign neoplasm
  - Lipomas: most are in the ileum, may cause obstruction
  - Hamartomas: part of Peutz-Jeghers syndrome, polypoid, may cause intermittent intussusception and bleeding
  - Hemangiomas: small and diffuse or large and isolated, can cause recurrent GI hemorrhage
  - Symptoms and signs: often asymptomatic or cause abdominal pain, GI bleeding, abdominal distention, abdominal tenderness
  - Contrast radiography or enteroclysis may show tumor as filling defect or mass lesion; CT scan with contrast may show mass

- **Differential Diagnosis**
  - Rule out malignant tumors

- **Treatment**
  - Benign tumors require no specific treatment if asymptomatic
  - Symptomatic lesions require resection or endoscopic excision
  - Prognosis: good after resection of benign lesions

- **Pearl**

Benign tumors require no specific treatment if asymptomatic.

Reference

Blanchard DK et al: Tumors of the small intestine. World J Surg 2000;24:421.

Small Intestine Tumors, Malignant

■ Essentials of Diagnosis

- Adenocarcinoma: 50% of cases; risk factors include Crohn disease, polyposis syndromes, villous adenomas
- Lymphoma: 15–20% of cases; most common is extranodal lymphoma
- Stromal tumors: 10–20% of cases; distinction between benign and malignant is difficult
- Metastatic tumors: affect small bowel by direct extension, carcinomatosis, or hematogenous spread
- Symptoms and signs include abdominal pain, GI bleeding, malabsorption (lymphoma), weight loss, abdominal distention, abdominal tenderness, palpable abdominal mass (stromal tumor)
- Imaging: adenocarcinoma: radiographic contrast study shows annular lesion with ulcerated mucosa, "apple core" appearance; CT scan detects metastases and allows staging; lymphoma: CT scan shows diffuse bowel wall thickening, mesenteric adenopathy, mass lesion; stromal tumors: CT scan shows extraluminal mass with vascularity and central necrosis

■ Differential Diagnosis

- Rule out benign tumors

■ Treatment

- All malignant tumors require wide segmental resection; even if not curative, resection may palliate obstruction and bleeding
- Prognosis: adenocarcinoma has 80% survival if localized, 10–15% if positive nodes; lymphoma 5-year survival is 20–40%; stromal tumors have 20% 5-year survival if high grade

■ Pearl

Always evaluate entire small bowel for synchronous lesions.

Reference

Cunningham JD et al: Malignant small bowel neoplasms: Histopathologic determinants of recurrence and survival. Ann Surg 1997;225:300.

Small Intestine, Infectious Diseases

- ■ Essentials of Diagnosis
  - Human immunodeficiency virus (HIV)-associated enteropathy: associated with opportunistic GI infections, intestinal perforation
  - *Yersinia* enteritis: associated with acute gastroenteritis, terminal ileitis, mesenteric lymphadenitis, hepatic and splenic abscesses
  - *Campylobacter jejuni* enteritis: from raw milk, untreated drinking water, or undercooked poultry
  - TB enteritis: most infections are due to swallowing the human tubercle bacillus
  - *Salmonella typhi*: may cause ulcers in distal ileum or cecum
  - Symptoms and signs include fever, diarrhea, chronic or relapsing bloody diarrhea in severe cases, nausea and vomiting, abdominal pain, abdominal tenderness

- ■ Differential Diagnosis
  - Pathogens involved in HIV-associated enteropathy include cryptosporidium, cytomegalovirus, *Entamoeba histolytica, Giardia lamblia,* mycobacterium avium-intracellulare, *Salmonella typhimurium, Shigella, C jejuni,* HIV
  - Rule out noninfectious causes of GI inflammation (pancreatitis, appendicitis)

- ■ Treatment
  - Appendectomy for symptoms and signs (usually presumed appendicitis) and if entire distal small bowel is grossly inflamed
  - Resection of small bowel is indicated for complications (obstruction, bleeding, perforation)

- ■ Pearl
  Careful hand washing limits nosocomial transmission.

Reference
Giannella RA: Enteric infections: 50 years of progress. Gastroenterology 1993;104:1589.

Small Intestine, Obstruction

- **Essentials of Diagnosis**
  - Adhesions: most common cause of mechanical obstruction
  - Hernia: due to incarceration of bowel
  - Neoplasms: intrinsic or extrinsic
  - Intussusception: common in children
  - Volvulus: from congenital anomalies or acquired adhesions
  - Foreign bodies: cause luminal blockage
  - Gallstone ileus: large gallstone in cholecystenteric fistula
  - Inflammatory bowel disease: luminal inflammation, fibrosis
  - Stricture: luminal narrowing
  - Cystic fibrosis: partial obstruction of distal ileum and right colon
  - Post-traumatic: hematoma of bowel wall or mesentery
  - Symptoms and signs include vomiting, cramping abdominal pain, obstipation; distention is minimal in proximal obstruction, pronounced in distal obstruction; mild abdominal tenderness; audible rushes and high-pitched tinkles; strangulation obstruction: shock, fever, abdominal tenderness and rigidity
  - Abdominal x-ray shows dilated bowel, air-fluid levels (minimal in early, proximal, or closed-loop obstruction); contrast upper GI series assesses completeness of obstruction; CT scan reveals intraperitoneal free fluid, dilated bowel proximal to and decompressed bowel distal to obstruction; point of obstruction may be visualized

- **Differential Diagnosis**
  - Acute appendicitis, gastroenteritis, pancreatitis
  - Obstruction of large intestine; mesenteric vascular occlusion

- **Treatment**
  - Partial obstruction: treat expectantly if continued passage of stool and flatus; successful in 90%; NG decompression
  - Surgical procedure varies by cause of obstruction; goals are relief of obstruction and correction of underlying cause
  - Surgery is indicated for persistent incomplete obstruction, complete obstruction, closed-loop obstruction, strangulation
  - Prognosis: mortality with nonstrangulating obstruction is about 2%; mortality with strangulating obstruction is 8–25%

- **Pearl**

Never let the sun set on a complete bowel obstruction.

Reference

Jenkins JT: Secondary causes of intestinal obstruction: Rigorous preoperative evaluation is required. Am Surg 2000;66:662.

Section V

Hepatobiliary Surgery

Chapters

19

Liver & Portal Venous System

Ascites

- ■ **Essentials of Diagnosis**
  - Causes include decreased plasma oncotic pressure (liver disease, malnutrition), increased lymph or peritoneal fluid production (liver disease, malignant ascites), blockage or disruption of abdominal lymphatic drainage (chylous ascites, congenital)
  - Symptoms and signs include abdominal distention or vague constitutional symptoms; ascites from cirrhosis associated with systemic signs of liver disease; malignant ascites associated with weight loss, a history of cancer, or symptoms related to the neoplasm
  - Liver failure causes hypoalbuminemia, increased prothrombin time, serum-ascites albumin gradient (SAAG) >1.1
  - Chylous ascites causes hypoalbuminemia, lymphocytopenia, anemia, SAAG <1.1
  - Malignant ascites causes positive tumor markers
  - Diagnostic tests include paracentesis for a positive cytologic diagnosis; abdominal/pelvic computed tomography (CT) scans for documenting ascites, suggesting liver disease, detecting lymphadenopathy and masses of the mesentery

- ■ **Differential Diagnosis**
  - Portal hypertension
  - Chylous ascites, malignant ascites
  - Biloma, urinoma
  - Soft-tissue neoplasm
  - Spontaneous bacterial peritonitis

- ■ **Treatment**
  - Medical management with diuretics, therapeutic paracentesis, and chemotherapy when indicated
  - Surgery: portovenous decompression in patients with good liver synthetic function; peritoneal-jugular shunt for refractory malignant ascites in selected patients
  - Medications include spironolactone with or without furosemide

- ■ **Pearl**

The best management for ascites is treatment of the underlying cause.

References

MELD (Model for End-Stage Liver Disease) Calculator. http://www.unos.org/resources/meldpeldcalculator.asp

Uriz J et al: Pathophysiology, diagnosis and treatment of ascites in cirrhosis. Baillieres Best Pract Res Clin Gastroenterol 2000;14:927.

Cirrhosis

- **Essentials of Diagnosis**
  - Develops in 15% of alcoholic patients; alcoholism is most common cause; other causes include idiopathic, viral hepatitis, hemochromatosis, Wilson disease, primary biliary cirrhosis, primary sclerosing cholangitis, Budd-Chiari syndrome, tricuspid regurgitation or stenosis, chronic allograft rejection in patients with liver transplant
  - Symptoms and signs include jaundice, ascites, bleeding varices, edema, spider angiomas, dark urine, light-colored stools, hyperbilirubinemia, hypoalbuminemia, prolonged prothrombin time, ascites on CT or ultrasound, hepatic fibrosis and nodularity on CT or ultrasound

- **Differential Diagnosis**
  - Cause (alcohol, virus, hemochromatosis, Wilson disease)
  - Hematoma
  - Gastrointestinal (GI) bleeding

- **Treatment**
  - Surgery: liver transplantation, transjugular intrahepatic portosystemic shunt (TIPS) versus surgical shunt for portal hypertension
  - Contraindications to liver transplantation: continued alcoholism, medical comorbid conditions
  - Medications: spironolactone, lactulose, β-blockers
  - Low-protein, low-salt diet
  - Prognosis: 30% mortality rate at 1 year after diagnosis, 50% mortality with variceal bleeding, 60–70% 5-year survival after liver transplantation

- **Pearl**

Diseases that cause cirrhosis in the first liver can do so in the second one also.

References

Kamath PS et al: A model to predict survival in patients with end-stage liver disease. Hepatology 2001;33:464.

MELD (Model for End-Stage Liver Disease) Calculator. http://www.unos.org/resources/meldpeldcalculator.asp

Cirrhosis, Primary Biliary

- **Essentials of Diagnosis**
  - Autoimmune disease characterized by portal tract inflammation
  - Symptoms and signs include increasing fatigue and pruritus; hyperbilirubinemia often evolves over 20 years
  - Workup: perform history and physical examination, CT of the abdomen, endoscopic retrograde cholangiopancreatography, liver function tests, anti–smooth muscle cell antibody, anti-mitochondrial antibody, liver biopsy

- **Differential Diagnosis**
  - Hepatitis
  - Biliary obstruction secondary to anatomic lesion

- **Treatment**
  - Liver transplantation is indicated for bilirubin >10 mg/dL
  - Prognosis: 60–70% 5-year survival after liver transplantation

- **Pearl**

Avoid procedures that would make the eventual liver transplantation more difficult.

References

MELD (Model for End-Stage Liver Disease) Calculator. http://www.unos.org/resources/meldpeldcalculator.asp

Talwalkar JA, Lindor KD: Primary biliary cirrhosis. Lancet 2003;362:53.

Hepatic Abscess

■ Essentials of Diagnosis

  • Causes include benign or malignant obstruction with cholangitis, extrahepatic abdominal sepsis, trauma or surgery to right upper quadrant, hepatic artery thrombosis or hepatic artery chemotherapy
  • Risk factors include metastatic cancer, diabetes, alcoholism
  • Symptoms and signs include fever, right upper quadrant pain, jaundice, leukocytosis
  • Ultrasound and CT show multifocal or unifocal hepatic abscesses, unilocular in appearance, with contrast enhancement peripherally by CT; perform CT-guided aspiration of abscess for culture

■ Differential Diagnosis

  • Parasitic diseases of liver
  • Hepatic tumor
  • Hepatic adenoma or focal nodular hyperplasia

■ Treatment

  • Surgery: perform CT-guided aspiration and drainage for abscesses >2–3 cm and fewer than 3 total abscesses; treat biliary obstruction if present
  • Give empiric antibiotic therapy to cover GI flora
  • Complications: recurrent abscess, liver failure, bile leak

■ Pearl

Cover with effective antibiotic therapy before drainage.

Reference

Johannsen EC et al: Pyogenic liver abscesses. Infect Dis Clin North Am 2000;14:47.

Hepatic Failure, Acute

■ **Essentials of Diagnosis**

- Acute hepatic injury causes sudden loss of hepatocytes because of toxins, ischemia, or inflammatory reaction
- Fulminant hepatic failure defined as onset of encephalopathy within 8 weeks of injury; causes include hepatitis viruses, cytomegalovirus (CMV), Epstein-Barr virus (EBV), varicella, herpes virus, toxins (acetaminophen and isoniazid most common), ischemia, fatty liver of pregnancy, Reye syndrome, Wilson disease, lymphoma, hereditary metabolic disorders
- Symptoms and signs include jaundice, right upper quadrant pain, bleeding, encephalopathy, hyperbilirubinemia, elevated transaminases, prolonged prothrombin time
- Workup should include history and physical examination; serum antibodies for hepatitis viruses, CMV, and EBV; ceruloplasmin level (Wilson disease)

■ **Differential Diagnosis**

- Hepatitis viruses, CMV, EBV, varicella, herpes virus
- Toxins (acetaminophen, isoniazid most common)
- Other causes: ischemia, fatty liver of pregnancy, Reye syndrome, Wilson disease, lymphoma, hereditary metabolic disorders

■ **Treatment**

- Liver transplantation is indicated for fulminant or subfulminant hepatic failure unresponsive to medical management
- Medications: N-acetylcysteine, minimize hypoglycemia, broad-spectrum antibiotics for any fever, fresh frozen plasma for planned invasive interventions
- Prognosis: 60–70% 5-year survival after liver transplantation; rapid disease onset is associated with more favorable prognosis

■ **Pearl**

Evaluate for transplant list early.

References

MELD (Model for End-Stage Liver Disease) Calculator. http://www.unos.org/resources/meldpeldcalculator.asp

Schiodt FV, Lee WM: Fulminant liver disease. Clin Liver Dis 2003;7:331.

Hepatic Neoplasms, Benign

- **Essentials of Diagnosis**
  - Most hepatic masses are benign; major diagnoses include adenoma, hemangioma, focal nodular hyperplasia, cysts, angiomyolipoma, regenerative nodules
  - Most masses are asymptomatic and seen on imaging studies performed for other reasons
  - Adenoma: homogeneous and hyperintense on T1- or T2-weighted magnetic resonance imaging (MRI) or CT, but 10–20% have hemorrhagic areas, making appearance heterogeneous
  - Hemangioma: early peripheral enhancement with intravenous (IV) contrast on CT, MRI, or tagged red cell scan
  - Focal nodular hyperplasia: CT or MRI shows stellate scar and enhancement with IV contrast
  - Cysts: hypointense or water density on ultrasound, CT, or MRI with no septations

- **Differential Diagnosis**
  - Adenoma, hemangioma, focal nodular hyperplasia, cysts, angiomyolipoma, regenerative nodules, abscess
  - Parasitic liver infection
  - Primary or metastatic malignancy

- **Treatment**
  - Perform surgical enucleation if diagnosis is secure, lesions are symptomatic, or adenomas are >5 cm; formal resection if diagnosis is in doubt
  - Discontinue estrogens or androgens for suspected adenomas, focal nodular hyperplasia, or hemangiomas

- **Pearl**

  Benign hepatic lesions can rupture if large.

References

National Comprehensive Cancer Network: Practice Guidelines. http://www.nccn.org
Terkivatan T et al: Indications and long-term outcome of treatment for benign hepatic tumors: A critical appraisal. Arch Surg 2001;136:1033.

Hepatic Tumors, Metastatic

- ■ Essentials of Diagnosis
  - Most common tumors of the liver; 90% with extrahepatic metastases; 20% of patients with metastatic colon cancer have metastasis to the liver
  - Symptoms and signs include weight loss, fatigue, fevers, right upper quadrant pain
  - Portography (or use of MRI) improves on sensitivity of CT for masses in liver
  - Workup: perform history and physical examination, CT with portography, MRI if CT is nondiagnostic

- ■ Differential Diagnosis
  - Rule out extrahepatic disease before considering resection

- ■ Treatment
  - Surgical resection
  - Hepatic artery chemotherapy (metastatic colon cancer only)
  - Radiofrequency ablation or cryotherapy for unresectable lesions if all can be addressed and extrahepatic disease is absent
  - Most common resectable tumors are colon, endocrine, melanoma
  - Contraindications to surgery: extrahepatic disease
  - Monitor treatment with carcinoembryonic antigen levels for colon cancer; CT scanning
  - Prognosis: colon cancer has 25% 5-year survival with resection

- ■ Pearl

Resection must be complete to be helpful.

References

Harmon KE et al: Benefits and safety of hepatic resection for colorectal metastases. Arch Surg 1999;177:402.

National Comprehensive Cancer Network: Practice Guidelines. http://www.nccn.org

Hepatic Tumor, Uncommon Primary

- ■ Essentials of Diagnosis
  - Tumors include angiosarcoma, hepatoblastoma, hepatic adeno-carcinoma, intrahepatic cholangiocarcinoma
  - Symptoms and signs include right upper quadrant pain, weight loss, hepatomegaly
  - CT scan shows hypervascular tumor for angiosarcoma; multi-septate cyst for adenocarcinoma
  - Workup: perform CT scan followed by resection for diagnosis and treatment

- ■ Differential Diagnosis
  - Metastatic carcinoma
  - Benign neoplasm
  - Other abdominal malignancy

- ■ Treatment
  - Surgical resection for localized tumor
  - Contraindications: poor liver function, extrahepatic disease, diffuse hepatic disease
  - Medications: chemotherapy for unresectable lesions
  - Prognosis: resectable cholangiocarcinoma has 5-year survival of 15–20%; angiosarcoma has very poor prognosis; hepatoblastoma has overall survival of 50%

- ■ Pearl

Complete resection is the only potentially curative option.

References

National Comprehensive Cancer Network: Practice Guidelines. http://www.nccn.org
Tagge EP et al: Resection, including transplantation, for hepatoblastoma and hepatocellular carcinoma: Impact on survival. J Pediatr Surg 1992;27:292.

Hepatitis (Acute & Chronic)

- ■ **Essentials of Diagnosis**
  - Virus is the most common cause; typically hepatitis B, C, and A
  - Symptoms and signs include right upper quadrant pain, jaundice, liver failure
  - Workup: perform history and physical examination, hepatic transaminases, anti-hepatitis B core antibody, surface antigen, anti-hepatitis B early antigen antibody, anti-hepatitis C antibody

- ■ **Differential Diagnosis**
  - Cholecystitis
  - Choledocholithiasis
  - Pancreatitis
  - Cholangitis

- ■ **Treatment**
  - Liver transplantation is indicated for fulminant liver failure, cirrhosis, hepatoma
  - Medications: interferon (for hepatitis B and C), ribavirin (for hepatitis C), anti-hepatitis A immunoglobulin, lamivudine (for chronic hepatitis B)
  - Prognosis: 90% remission or recovery in hepatitis B; 10% have chronic hepatitis B (70–90% as carrier only); 55–70% have chronic hepatitis C

- ■ **Pearl**

Hepatitis B is a major preventable occupational risk to health care workers.

References

Centers for Disease Control and Prevention: http://www.cdc.gov

MELD (Model for End-Stage Liver Disease) Calculator. http://www.unos.org/resources/meldpeldcalculator.asp

Hepatocellular Carcinoma

- **Essentials of Diagnosis**
  - 80% of primary hepatic malignancies; 50% with fibrous capsule; 70% with extrahepatic disease
  - Metastases most common to hilar and celiac nodes
  - Associated with all causes of cirrhosis
  - Greatest incidence in Asia and Africa
  - Symptoms and signs include right upper quadrant pain, weight loss, jaundice, hepatomegaly
  - CT with IV portography often shows hypervascular tumor, frequently with multicentric disease; ultrasound shows hyperechoic tumor; combination of CT, ultrasound, and MRI is 80% sensitive
  - Tumor marker: serum alpha-fetoprotein

- **Differential Diagnosis**
  - Metastatic hepatic carcinoma
  - Cholangiocarcinoma
  - Benign neoplasm
  - Other abdominal malignancy

- **Treatment**
  - Liver transplantation is treatment of choice in the presence of cirrhosis; partial hepatectomy with at least 0.5-cm margins (25% are candidates)
  - Contraindications: medical comorbidity, total tumor volume >6.5 cm (for liver transplantation)
  - Ablative procedures: ethyl alcohol ablation (75% complete necrosis), radiofrequency ablation
  - Prognosis: after resection, 5-year survival for noncirrhotic is 40%, 5-year survival for fibrolamellar is 60%; after transplantation, 5-year survival is 70%

- **Pearl**

Transplantation addresses the field defect in cirrhotic patients with hepatocellular carcinoma.

References

Akriviadis EA et al: Hepatocellular carcinoma. Br J Surg 1998;85:1319.

MELD (Model for End-Stage Liver Disease) Calculator. http://www.unos.org/resources/meldpeldcalculator.asp

National Comprehensive Cancer Network: Practice Guidelines. http://www.nccn.org

Portal Hypertension

- ### Essentials of Diagnosis
  - Causes include cirrhosis, congenital hepatic fibrotic disorders, acute liver failure, Budd-Chiari syndrome
  - Bleeding gastroesophageal varices are most important complication; varices are related to degree of liver dysfunction
  - Symptoms and signs include hematemesis, melena, jaundice, encephalopathy
  - CT scan shows dilated venous collaterals, possible venous thrombosis; ultrasound shows dilated portal vein, possible thrombosis of portal vein or hepatic veins; esophagogastroscopy for diagnosis of varices

- ### Differential Diagnosis
  - Check for other sources of upper GI bleeding using esophagogastroscopy

- ### Treatment
  - Sclerotherapy or banding of varices (by esophagogastroscopy), TIPS, Sengstaken-Blakemore tube placement, blood products as necessary
  - Surgery: liver transplantation; surgical portosystemic shunt (TIPS vs total vs partial vs selective)
  - Liver transplantation is indicated if donor is available, no medical comorbidity, not currently drinking alcohol
  - Surgical shunt is indicated for Childs A failed endoscopic therapy, elective (selective) or emergent (partial)
  - Medications: β-blockers, nitrates, vasopressin (during bleeding), octreotide (during bleeding)
  - Complications: encephalopathy (for shunts), hemorrhage, shunt thrombosis; survival is related to MELD (Model for End-Stage Liver Disease) or Child class

- ### Pearl

Morbidity of extrahepatic abdominal procedures is increased in patients with portal hypertension.

References

Krige JE, Beckingham IJ: ABC of diseases of liver, pancreas, and biliary system. Portal hypertension-1: Varices. BMJ 2001;322:348.

Krige JE, Beckingham IJ: ABC of diseases of liver, pancreas, and biliary system. Portal hypertension-2: Ascites, encephalopathy, and other conditions. BMJ 2001;322:416.

MELD (Model for End-Stage Liver Disease) Calculator. http://www.unos.org/resources/meldpeldcalculator.asp

Splenic Vein Thrombosis

- **Essentials of Diagnosis**
  - Upper GI hemorrhage with evidence of gastric varices without esophageal varices; history of pancreatic or gastric disease; isolated thrombosis in the splenic vein, diverting the splenic venous outflow to the short gastric vessels as collaterals
  - 50% of cases are due to pancreatitis or pancreatic pseudocyst; pancreatic cancer with splenic vein invasion is the second most common cause
  - Symptoms and signs include upper GI hemorrhage, possible splenomegaly
  - Gastroscopy shows bleeding as evidence of gastric varices, without evidence of esophageal varices; also perform upper GI endoscopy

- **Differential Diagnosis**
  - Portal hypertension
  - Other sources of upper GI bleeding

- **Treatment**
  - Splenectomy is curative and indicated in all cases
  - Even if patient is asymptomatic and has not experienced upper GI bleeding, splenectomy should be performed electively

- **Pearl**

Splenic vein thrombosis is the most easily correctable cause of variceal bleeding.

Reference

Loftus JP et al: Sinistral portal hypertension. Splenectomy or expectant management. Ann Surg 1993;217:35.

20

Biliary Tract

Ampulla of Vater Tumors

■ Essentials of Diagnosis

- Partial or complete obstruction of the common bile duct and pancreatic duct at the ampulla of Vater
- Of primary tumors of the ampulla of Vater, 33% are adenomas and 67% are adenocarcinomas
- Symptoms and signs include jaundice, abdominal pain, and weight loss as presenting symptoms; gastrointestinal (GI) bleeding from ampullary tumor; elevated serum bilirubin
- Computed tomography (CT) scan shows dilatation of the biliary tree and pancreatic duct and is also used for staging; endoscopic retrograde cholangiopancreatography (ERCP) shows dilatation of the biliary and pancreatic ducts; endoscopy shows exophytic mass at the ampulla

■ Differential Diagnosis

- If a tumor of the ampulla of Vater is suspected but not visualized on duodenoscopy, sphincterotomy should be performed to inspect the intraluminal surface of the ampulla
- Rule out benign causes of biliary obstruction, cholangiocarcinoma, pancreatic adenocarcinoma, duodenal adenoma or adenocarcinoma

■ Treatment

- All ampullary adenomas and adenocarcinomas should be resected
- Adenomas: local excision or pancreaticoduodenectomy
- Adenocarcinomas: pancreaticoduodenectomy
- Contraindications to resection: distant metastases (hepatic)
- Prognosis: 5-year survival after resection of adenocarcinoma is 50%

■ Pearl

Fifty percent of ampullary adenomas contain carcinoma in the resection specimen despite benign preoperative biopsy.

References

Howe JR et al: Factors predictive of survival in ampullary carcinoma. Ann Surg 1998;228:87.
National Comprehensive Cancer Network: Practice Guidelines. http://www.nccn.org

Biliary Neoplasms, Benign

- ■ Essentials of Diagnosis
  - Gallbladder adenoma: rare, considered a premalignant lesion
  - Papillomatosis: multiple gallbladder adenomas
  - Adenomyomatosis: gallbladder wall hyperplasia that can be diffuse, possibly premalignant
  - Other possible benign biliary neoplasms: leiomyomas, lipomas, hemangiomas, and heterotopic GI tissue
  - Benign biliary neoplasms may be asymptomatic or cause biliary colic, cholecystitis, jaundice, hyperbilirubinemia
  - Right upper quadrant ultrasound shows thickened gallbladder wall for adenomyomatosis, submuscular hyperechoic areas for cholesterol polyps, biliary dilatation and possible stricture for benign biliary neoplasms
  - Measure carcinoembryonic antigen and CA 19-9; perform right upper quadrant ultrasound, percutaneous transhepatic cholangiography (PTC), or ERCP

- ■ Differential Diagnosis
  - Rule out malignancy
  - Resection is often necessary to verify diagnosis

- ■ Treatment
  - Cholecystectomy for gallbladder adenomatous polyps >1 cm
  - Resection of biliary stricture and bilioenteric reconstruction for benign biliary neoplasms causing jaundice or cholangitis, biliary leak, or stricture

- ■ Pearl

Resection is often necessary to rule out early malignancy.

References

Doherty GM, Way LW: Biliary tract. In Way LW, Doherty GM (editors): Current Surgical Diagnosis & Treatment, 11th ed. McGraw-Hill, 2003.
National Comprehensive Cancer Network: Practice Guidelines. http://www.nccn.org

Biliary Obstruction, Benign

■ **Essentials of Diagnosis**

- Causes include postoperative, trauma, chronic pancreatitis, cholelithiasis or choledocholithiasis, primary sclerosing cholangitis, sphincter of Oddi stenosis, duodenal ulcer, Crohn disease, viral infection, drug toxins
- Symptoms and signs include fever, abdominal pain, jaundice, hyperbilirubinemia
- Right upper quadrant ultrasound shows associated biloma with postoperative stricture, biliary dilatation, atrophic or calcified pancreas; magnetic resonance cholangiopancreatography (MRCP) or PTC helpful to evaluate biliary tree; endoscopic ultrasound to evaluate possible pancreatic head mass

■ **Differential Diagnosis**

- Rule out biliary, pancreatic, or ampullary malignancy

■ **Treatment**

- Hepaticojejunostomy for most postoperative or traumatic strictures
- Choledochoduodenostomy or choledochojejunostomy for chronic, pancreatitis-induced strictures
- Balloon dilation indicated for some anastomotic biliary strictures after repair
- Complications: recurrent stricture, biliary leak
- Prognosis: excellent in 70–90% after surgical reconstruction; poor for balloon dilation as primary therapy for strictures, except as treatment for early post-repair stricture

■ **Pearl**

Allow acute inflammation to resolve before attempting any definitive repair.

Reference

Nealon WH, Urrutia F: Long-term follow-up after bilioenteric anastomosis for benign bile duct stricture. Ann Surg 1996;223:639.

Cholangiocarcinoma

- **Essentials of Diagnosis**
  - Arises from biliary epithelium; risk factors include primary sclerosing cholangitis, choledochal cysts, *Clonorchis* infection
  - Symptoms and signs include painless jaundice, right upper quadrant pain, pruritus, anorexia, malaise, weight loss, hyperbilirubinemia, elevated alkaline phosphatase, elevated CA 19-9
  - Ultrasound shows dilated extrahepatic and intrahepatic biliary ducts (depending on level of tumor); PTC or MRCP shows proximal and distal extent of tumor; PTC allows brushings for cytologic studies of tumor
  - CA 19-9 is a useful tumor marker
  - Workup: perform ultrasound to screen for anatomic causes of hyperbilirubinemia, abdominal CT, PTC, or MRCP (PTC if brushings are needed)

- **Differential Diagnosis**
  - Extrahepatic disease or bilobar involvement
  - Choledocholithiasis

- **Treatment**
  - Biliary resection followed by biliary-enteric reconstruction
  - Extended right or left lobectomy if proximal disease noted (isolated to 1 side) above secondary radicals or if unilateral portal vein involvement
  - Pancreaticoduodenectomy (Whipple) for tumors of the distal common bile duct (CBD)
  - Indications for operation: resectable cholangiocarcinoma versus benign stricture can be difficult to distinguish
  - Contraindications: bilobar involvement or second-order biliary radicals bilaterally
  - Prognosis: 10–30% 5-year survival with curative resection of proximal biliary tumor; 30–50% 5-year survival with distal CBD tumor

- **Pearl**

The best opportunity for cure is initial operation; do not miss this by assuming a patient with obstructive jaundice has choledocholithiasis.

References

Jarnagin WR: Cholangiocarcinoma of the extrahepatic bile ducts. Semin Surg Oncol 2000;19:156.

National Comprehensive Cancer Network: Practice Guidelines. http://www.nccn.org

Cholangitis, Primary Sclerosing

- ■ Essentials of Diagnosis
  - • Associated with ulcerative colitis in 40–60%, pancreatitis in 12–25%, diabetes mellitus in 5–10%, and rarely other autoimmune disorders
  - • Increased risk for cholangiocarcinoma
  - • Symptoms and signs include intermittent jaundice, fever, right upper quadrant pain, pruritus, elevated alkaline phosphatase, hyperbilirubinemia
  - • Right upper quadrant ultrasound, ERCP, and MRCP may show multiple dilations and strictures of extrahepatic biliary ducts; perform abdominal ultrasound, ERCP, or liver biopsy if question of cirrhosis; obtain brushings by PTC or ERCP if question of malignancy

- ■ Differential Diagnosis
  - • Cholangiocarcinoma
  - • Cirrhosis
  - • Choledocholithiasis

- ■ Treatment
  - • Balloon dilation of multiple strictures
  - • Resection of dominant stricture followed by biliary reconstruction
  - • Liver transplantation (preferably before onset of cirrhosis)
  - • Prognosis: 85% survival rate 5 years after transplantation; 71% actuarial survival at 5 years after resection of dominant stricture (only 20% if cirrhosis present); 43% long-term success with balloon therapy for multiple strictures

- ■ Pearl
  Early liver transplantation saves lives and effort.

Reference

Kim WR et al: A revised natural history model for primary sclerosing cholangitis. Mayo Clin Proc 2000;75:688.

Cholecystitis (Acute & Chronic)

- ■ Essentials of Diagnosis
  - Cholesterol stones form in 20% of women and 10% of men by age 60 years
  - Risk factors include female gender, age, obesity, estrogen exposure, fatty diet, rapid weight loss
  - Symptoms develop in about 3% of asymptomatic patients each year (20–30% over 20 years)
  - Acalculous cholecystitis affects patients with acute, severe systemic illness
  - Symptoms and signs include unremitting biliary colic in epigastrium or right upper quadrant, fever, nausea, vomiting, right upper quadrant pain to palpation with peritoneal signs, Murphy sign, anorexia, leukocytosis
  - Right upper quadrant ultrasound shows gallstones, gallbladder wall thickening (>4 mm), or pericholecystic fluid (no stones if acalculous cholecystitis); hepato-iminodiacetic acid (HIDA) scan shows failure of gallbladder filling (>95% sensitive); CT shows gallbladder wall thickening (>4 mm) and pericholecystic fluid in patients with suspected acalculous cholecystitis as sensitively as ultrasound
  - Perform complete blood count, amylase and lipase, right upper quadrant ultrasound, HIDA scan for difficult cases

- ■ Differential Diagnosis
  - Choledocholithiasis
  - Pancreatitis

- ■ Treatment
  - All patients require intravenous fluids and antibiotics, followed by early cholecystectomy (preferred) or cholecystectomy after about 6 weeks if acute episode resolves with antibiotics
  - Delayed strategy is most helpful in patients who present after acute episode has gone on for a few days; late presentation makes early cholecystectomy more difficult and complicated
  - Surgery includes laparoscopic or open cholecystectomy; cholecystectomy tube (if cholecystectomy too hazardous)

- ■ Pearl

Patients at risk: fair, fat, forty, fertile, and female.

References

Berber E et al: Selective use of tube cholecystostomy with interval laparoscopic cholecystectomy in acute cholecystitis. Arch Surg 2000;135:341.

Svanvik J: Laparoscopic cholecystectomy for acute cholecystitis. Eur J Surg 2000(suppl 585):16.

Choledochal Cyst

- ■ Essentials of Diagnosis
    - Type I cyst (fusiform dilatation of CBD) accounts for 85–90%; type II (true diverticula of CBD) in 1–2%; type III (choledochocele; dilatation of distal CBD) in 2%; type IV (multiple cysts involving intrahepatic and extrahepatic ducts) as high as 15% of cases in some series; type V (cystic malformation of intrahepatic ducts) is rare; 3–5% incidence of carcinoma within cyst
    - Symptoms and signs include jaundice, fever, pain, hyperbilirubinemia
    - Ultrasound shows characteristic cystic dilatation of biliary tree corresponding to type, as well as proximal dilatation in presence of obstruction
    - Perform liver function tests, abdominal ultrasound, ERCP or MRCP (adults)

- ■ Differential Diagnosis
    - Choledocholithiasis
    - Cholecystitis
    - Intestinal duplication
    - Primary sclerosing cholangitis

- ■ Treatment
    - Types I–III: cyst excision and biliary reconstruction
    - Types IV and V: treatment is individualized and may require partial hepatectomy for unilobar involvement
    - Surveillance for carcinoma because patients are still at increased risk for remainder of biliary tree

- ■ Pearl

Thorough preoperative imaging is necessary for operative planning.

Reference

Vercruysse R, Van den Bossche MR: Choledochal cyst in adults. Acta Chir Belg 1998;98:220.

Choledocholithiasis & Gallstone Pancreatitis

- ■ Essentials of Diagnosis
  - Cholesterol stone risk factors include female gender, age, obesity, estrogen exposure, fatty diet, rapid weight loss
  - Complicated gallstone disease affects <0.5% of asymptomatic patients annually
  - Patients may be asymptomatic, or symptoms and signs may include right upper quadrant pain, painless jaundice, fever, conjugated hyperbilirubinemia (for choledocholithiasis), elevated alkaline phosphatase (for choledocholithiasis), leukocytosis (for pancreatitis or cholangitis)
  - Right upper quadrant ultrasound shows gallstones, dilated CBD (>6 mm), and CBD stones in only 20–30% of patients with choledocholithiasis; ERCP shows dilated CBD and single or multiple CBD stones in patients with choledocholithiasis
  - Workup: perform liver function tests, amylase and lipase, right upper quadrant ultrasound, ERCP or laparoscopic cholangiography

- ■ Differential Diagnosis
  - Rule out biliary stricture

- ■ Treatment
  - Strategy should reflect patient's status and the expertise and preferences of surgeon and biliary gastroenterologist
  - ERCP with sphincterotomy and stone extraction followed by laparoscopic cholecystectomy
  - Laparoscopic cholecystectomy with CBD exploration
  - Laparoscopic cholecystectomy and stone extraction
  - Indications for operation include choledocholithiasis (symptomatic or asymptomatic) and gallstone pancreatitis
  - Prognosis: gallstone pancreatitis resolves in >90% of cases

- ■ Pearl

Patients at risk: fair, fat, forty, fertile, and female.

Reference

Rosenthal RJ et al: Options and strategies for the management of choledocholithiasis. World J Surg 1998;22:1125.

Cholelithiasis

- **Essentials of Diagnosis**
    - Divided into symptomatic and asymptomatic; caused by cholesterol (most common), black pigment, or brown pigment stones
    - Cholesterol stones form in 20% of women and 10% of men by age 60 years
    - Overall risk factors include female gender, age, obesity, estrogen exposure, fatty diet, rapid weight loss
    - Black pigment stone risk factors include hemolytic disorders, living in Asia
    - Brown pigment stone risk factors include biliary stasis, biliary infections
    - Each year, complicated gallstone disease affects 3–5% of patients who are symptomatic and <0.5% of patients who are asymptomatic
    - Symptoms and signs range from asymptomatic to biliary colic
    - Right upper quadrant ultrasound shows acoustically dense stones in gallbladder
    - Evaluate amylase and lipase; perform right upper quadrant ultrasound

- **Differential Diagnosis**
    - Cholecystitis
    - Choledocholithiasis
    - Pancreatitis

- **Treatment**
    - Laparoscopic cholecystectomy for symptomatic cholelithiasis or porcelain gallbladder (25% risk of carcinoma)

- **Pearl**

Patients at risk: fair, fat, forty, fertile, and female.

Reference

Fletcher DR et al: Complications of cholecystectomy: Risks of the laparoscopic approach and protective effects of operative cholangiography: A population-based study. Ann Surg 1999;229:449.

Cholelithiasis, Rare Complications

- ■ Essentials of Diagnosis
  - Gallstone ileus: small bowel obstruction secondary to 1 or more large gallstones entering via cholecystoduodenal fistula
  - Mirizzi syndrome: biliary stricture secondary to direct compression by chronically impacted cystic duct gallstone or chronically inflamed gallbladder
  - Epidemiology: both gallstone ileus and Mirizzi syndrome are rare, mainly affecting patients >60 years
  - Imaging findings in gallstone ileus: abdominal x-ray shows air-fluid levels, dilated loops of small bowel, possible pneumobilia; ultrasound shows cholelithiasis and pneumobilia; swallow study with water-soluble contrast shows fistula between duodenum and gallbladder
  - Imaging findings in Mirizzi syndrome: ultrasound shows biliary dilatation (>6 mm), cholelithiasis, possible thickened wall of gallbladder
  - Workup: for gallstone ileus, obtain plain abdominal x-ray, right upper quadrant ultrasound, small bowel contrast study if partial small bowel obstruction; for Mirizzi syndrome, perform liver function tests, right upper quadrant ultrasound

- ■ Differential Diagnosis
  - Cholecystitis, choledocholithiasis, choledochal cyst
  - Hepatitis
  - Pancreatitis
  - Adhesive bowel obstruction

- ■ Treatment
  - Gallstone ileus: remove retained small bowel gallstone(s) via enterostomy or partial resection if bowel is ischemic; perform cholecystectomy and resection of fistula plus duodenal closure at same operation or as staged procedure
  - Mirizzi syndrome: perform cholecystectomy and resection or bypass of stricture via hepaticojejunostomy

- ■ Pearl

These rare complications are more common in elderly patients.

Reference

Doherty GM, Way LW: Biliary tract. In Way LW, Doherty GM (editors): Current Surgical Diagnosis & Treatment, 11th ed. McGraw-Hill, 2003.

Gallbladder Adenocarcinoma

- ■ Essentials of Diagnosis
  - Risk factors include gallstones (70–90% of patients), Native American heritage, stones >3 cm (10-fold increased risk), porcelain gallbladder (≥25% develop cancer), choledochal cyst, gallbladder adenoma >1 cm
  - Incidence: 3:1 female to male ratio; peak incidence in seventh decade; risk is at least 5% among Native Americans with gallstones
  - Symptoms and signs include biliary colic or cholecystitis, jaundice, weight loss, hyperbilirubinemia, elevated alkaline phosphatase, elevated carcinoembryonic antigen
  - Right upper quadrant ultrasound shows gallbladder inflammation, gallstones, or both; occasional gallbladder mass; CT or MRI shows gallbladder mass (90% sensitive) with occasional portal lymphadenopathy; hepatic extension of tumor

- ■ Differential Diagnosis
  - Lymph node involvement
  - Extension into extrahepatic biliary tree
  - Extension into hepatic parenchyma

- ■ Treatment
  - Cholecystectomy (for T1 tumors, limited to muscular wall)
  - Cholecystectomy with segment 4b, 5 liver resection and portal lymphadenectomy (for T2 tumors, invasion to perimuscular tissue but not to serosa)
  - Right extended hepatectomy and resection of CBD followed by hepaticojejunostomy (for invasion into CBD or liver; T3 tumors)
  - Prognosis: 5% overall survival, 17% 5-year survival with resection for curative intent, >95% survival for T1 tumors treated with cholecystectomy, 70% to >90% survival for T2 and T3 tumors if at least 4b and 5 segment resections are performed and no nodal involvement

- ■ Pearl

Resection is the only chance for cure.

References

Baillie J: Tumors of the gallbladder and bile ducts. J Clin Gastroenterol 1999;29:14.

National Comprehensive Cancer Network: Practice Guidelines. http://www.nccn.org

Hepatobiliary Infections, Parasitic

- ■ Essentials of Diagnosis
  - Causes include amebic, echinococcal, schistosomal; hydatid cysts occur in liver (50–70% of cases) and lung (20–30% of cases); schistosomal infection is major cause of portal hypertension worldwide
  - Symptoms and signs include fever, right upper quadrant pain, jaundice
  - Laboratory tests show leukocytosis, elevated alkaline phosphatase, elevated transaminases; *Entamoeba histolytica* serologic studies are positive in 95% of cases of amebic abscess; hydatid serologic studies are positive in >80% of cases; schistosomal ova are found in feces; eosinophilia in hydatid disease
  - CT scan and ultrasound for amebic abscess show unifocal or multifocal fluid-filled areas in liver with peripheral contrast enhancement (not distinguishable from pyogenic)
  - CT scan for hydatid cyst shows daughter cysts within parent cyst accompanied by calcification

- ■ Differential Diagnosis
  - Pyogenic abscess
  - Hepatic tumor

- ■ Treatment
  - CT-guided drainage of hydatid cysts
  - Metronidazole with or without chloroquine for amebic abscess
  - Albendazole for 8 weeks for hydatid disease
  - Praziquantel for schistosomiasis

- ■ Pearl

Cover with effective antiparasitic agents before draining (and potentially spilling) cyst contents.

Reference

Doherty GM, Way LW: Liver & portal venous system. In Way LW, Doherty GM (editors): Current Surgical Diagnosis & Treatment, 11th ed. McGraw-Hill, 2003.

Jaundice

- **Essentials of Diagnosis**
  - Classified as obstructive (conjugated bilirubinemia) or nonobstructive (unconjugated bilirubinemia)
  - Causes in adults include obstruction from benign or malignant causes (stones, tumors, strictures), sludge or stasis due to infection or total parenteral nutrition (TPN), hemolysis, or hepatocellular dysfunction
  - Causes in neonates include physiologic, biliary atresia, choledochal cyst, TPN, hemolysis, Alagille syndrome, intrahepatic bile duct paucity, Byler syndrome
  - Symptoms and signs include jaundice, malaise, anorexia, hyperbilirubinemia (conjugated or unconjugated)
  - Ultrasound shows biliary dilatation if obstruction present; CT shows biliary obstruction and accompanying mass; ERCP, MRCP, and PTC show biliary obstruction if mass is present and distal extent

- **Differential Diagnosis**
  - Rule out anatomical obstruction to bile flow

- **Treatment**
  - Resolution of biliary tract stone disease by cholecystectomy and decompression of CBD by operative, radiologic, or endoscopic intervention
  - Resection of mass causing obstruction; biliary reconstruction
  - Other treatments: ursodiol, phototherapy (for neonates), exchange transfusion (neonates)
  - Monitor treatment with serum bilirubin

- **Pearl**

Evaluate for prehepatic, hepatic, and posthepatic causes.

Reference

Doherty GM, Way LW: Biliary tract. In Way LW, Doherty GM, (editors): Current Surgical Diagnosis & Treatment, 11th ed. McGraw-Hill, 2003.

Section VI

Lower Gastrointestinal Surgery

Chapters

21

Colon

Colitis, Antibiotic-Associated

- **Essentials of Diagnosis**
    - Diarrhea with or without gross mucosal abnormalities; also referred to as pseudomembranous colitis
    - Results from antibiotic therapy or alteration in colonic flora; clindamycin, ampicillin, cephalosporins are common inciting antibiotics; caused by *Clostridium difficile* toxins A and B
    - Symptoms and signs include watery, green diarrhea, sometimes bloody; complications including toxic megacolon or perforation may lead to peritoneal signs
    - Endoscopy (sigmoidoscopy) shows elevated plaques, pseudomembranes; erythematous, edematous mucosa

- **Differential Diagnosis**
    - Malignancy
    - Stricture
    - Ischemic colitis
    - Diverticulitis
    - Cholecystitis
    - Gastroenteritis
    - Peritonitis

- **Treatment**
    - Discontinue inciting antibiotic; give oral vancomycin for 7–10 days; oral metronidazole for 7–14 days; avoid antidiarrheal medications
    - Surgery indications: failure of medical management with worsening clinical course or progression to toxic megacolon, peritonitis, perforation
    - Prevention: proper hand washing and protective barrier (gown and gloves) with infected patients; discontinue unnecessary antibiotics
    - Prognosis: recurrence rate after treatment is 20%

- **Pearl**

Colitis can become apparent long after the antibiotics have been stopped.

Reference

Kelly CP et al: Clostridium difficile colitis. N Engl J Med 1994;330:257.

Colitis, Ischemic

- ■ Essentials of Diagnosis
  - Most common form of gastrointestinal (GI) ischemia; may occur after low-flow states: shock, myocardial infarction, abdominal aortic aneurysm repair
  - Symptoms and signs include abrupt onset of abdominal pain, diarrhea (may be bloody), fever, pain out of proportion to examination findings
  - Abdominal x-rays are nonspecific; computed tomography (CT) may show thickened bowel wall; colonoscopy may reveal edematous, hemorrhagic mucosa with or without ulcerations; grayish membrane resembles pseudomembranous colitis
  - Consider workup for hypercoagulable state, embolic source (transesophageal echocardiography, aortography)

- ■ Differential Diagnosis
  - Colorectal cancer
  - Diverticulitis
  - Inflammatory bowel disease
  - Pseudomembranous colitis
  - Infectious colitis

- ■ Treatment
  - Intravenous (IV) hydration, broad-spectrum antibiotics, bowel rest
  - Operative indications: irreversible disease, failure of conservative measures, full-thickness necrosis, stricture or obstruction
  - Complications: severe ischemic disease, ischemic stricture often associated with other comorbid conditions
  - Prognosis: overall mortality rate is ~50%

- ■ Pearl

The watershed area between the superior mesenteric artery distribution and the inferior mesenteric artery distribution is most sensitive to low-flow ischemia.

Reference

Hwang RF, Schwartz RW: Ischemic colitis: A brief review. Curr Surg 2001;58:192.

Colitis, Ulcerative

- ### Essentials of Diagnosis
  - Diffuse inflammatory disease confined to mucosa and submucosa; crypts of Lieberkühn abscesses; diseased areas are contiguous; increase in colorectal cancer risk
  - Symptoms and signs include rectal bleeding, diarrhea, tenesmus, rectal urgency
  - Sigmoidoscopy shows loss of normal vascular pattern; friable, hyperemic rectal mucosa; mucosal granularity; ulcers with bleeding and purulent exudates in advanced disease

- ### Differential Diagnosis
  - No radiographic, histologic, or endoscopic findings are pathognomonic
  - Rule out infectious diarrhea (shigellosis, salmonellosis, *Escherichia coli* infection, amebiasis), Crohn disease, malignancy, diverticular disease, *C difficile* colitis

- ### Treatment
  - Initially, medical unless complications arise; surgery is potentially curative; treatment focuses on containing and reducing inflammation
  - Medications include sulfasalazine, corticosteroids, mesalamine; cyclosporine for steroid-resistant colitis
  - Surgery: total colectomy, rectal mucosectomy, and ileoanal anastomosis; emergent procedures should be tailored to fit extent of the illness; typically total abdominal colectomy and ileostomy
  - Indications: emergency surgery for perforation; urgent surgery for medically refractory toxic megacolon, massive hemorrhage, fulminant acute flare unresponsive to medication
  - Prognosis: mortality declining over last 2 decades; 1–2% per year colorectal cancer risk

- ### Pearl
Some patients with severe toxic colitis are too sick not *to operate on.*

References

Crohn's and Colitis Foundation of America: http://www.ccfa.org
Eaden JA et al: The risk of colorectal cancer in ulcerative colitis: A meta-analysis. Gut 2001;48:526.

Colorectal Adenocarcinoma

- ■ Essentials of Diagnosis
  - Risk factors include ulcerative colitis, Crohn colitis, schistosomal colitis, exposure to radiation, ureterocolostomy
  - Distribution of colorectal cancer: 25% right colon, 10% transverse colon, 15% left colon, 20–50% rectosigmoid colon
  - Symptoms and signs: right colon lesions may become large before symptoms develop; may cause occult bleeding, anemia; left colon lesions often cause crampy abdominal pain; large bowel obstruction in 10% of cases
  - Total colonoscopy performed to evaluate lesion and detect synchronous lesions; CT scan is helpful to assess extramural extension or metastatic lesions; endorectal ultrasound determines depth of invasion of rectal lesions

- ■ Differential Diagnosis
  - Ulcerative colitis, Crohn colitis, ischemic colitis
  - Parasitic infection, amebiasis
  - Diverticulitis

- ■ Treatment
  - Resection of lesion and regional lymphatic drainage basin; adherent visceral structures resected en bloc; margins should be at least 2 cm
  - Rectal cancer: type of operation (abdominoperineal resection vs low anterior resection) determined by ability to achieve adequate margins (≥ 2 cm); right-sided lesions: resection includes distal ileum, ileocolic, right colic, and middle colic vessels; transverse colon lesions: transverse or extended right colectomy; left-sided lesions: inferior mesenteric artery
  - Preoperative radiotherapy increases 5-year survival and decreases local recurrence in rectal cancer; postoperative chemotherapy (5-fluorouracil) and radiation beneficial for stage II rectal cancer
  - Colon cancer: efficacy of chemotherapy is unclear for stage II; oral levamisole and IV 5-fluorouracil may be useful in stage III
  - Prognosis: 5-year survival rates are 80% for stage I, 60% for stage II, 30% for stage III, 5% for stage IV; 90% of recurrences occur within first 4 years after surgery

- ■ Pearl

Complete operative resection is the most important feature in potentially curative colorectal cancer treatment.

Reference

National Comprehensive Cancer Network: Practice Guidelines. http://www.nccn.org

Colorectal Cancer, Hereditary Nonpolyposis (HNPCC)

- ■ Essentials of Diagnosis
  - · 6% of patients with cancer of the colon or rectum have HNPCC
  - · Gene localized to chromosome 2p; Lynch syndrome II: early onset (average age 44 years), proximal dominance; Lynch syndrome I: hereditary site-specific colon cancer shows the same characteristics except no extracolonic cancers
  - · Diagnostic (Amsterdam) criteria: families must have at least 3 relatives with colorectal cancer, 1 of whom is a first-degree relative of the other 2; colorectal cancer involves at least 2 generations; and at least 1 cancer case occurs before age 50
  - · Alterations in DNA mismatch repair genes that help maintain DNA fidelity during replication are characteristic of HNPCC: *hMLH1*, *hPMS1* and *hPMS2*, and *hMSH6*
  - · Symptoms and signs: most patients are asymptomatic; lower GI bleeding may occur, although most bleeding is occult
  - · Mainstay of diagnosis of Lynch syndromes is a detailed family history; when a pedigree is identified, genetic counseling should be provided to decide about testing for genetic markers

- ■ Differential Diagnosis
  - · Always evaluate for synchronous colon carcinoma

- ■ Treatment
  - · When colon cancer is detected, abdominal colectomy with ileorectal anastomosis is the procedure of choice
  - · For women with no further plans for childbearing, prophylactic total abdominal hysterectomy and bilateral salpingo-oophorectomy are recommended
  - · Prevention: patients with a family history of HNPCC should have colonoscopy every 1–2 years beginning at age 20–30, then annually after age 40; prophylactic colectomy for patients with HNPCC is still controversial, although most experts now favor it

- ■ Pearl

Always refer inherited cancer syndrome patients to genetic counseling for personal and family evaluation, documentation, and follow-up.

References

Lynch HY, de la Chapelle A: Hereditary colorectal cancer. N Engl J Med 2003;348:919.

National Comprehensive Cancer Network: Practice Guidelines. http://www.nccn.org

Colorectal Tumors, Uncommon

- **Essentials of Diagnosis**
  - Carcinoids: uncommon in large bowel; most occur in rectum; carcinoid syndrome appears in <5% of patients with metastatic carcinoid of the large bowel; 60% of rectal carcinoids present as asymptomatic submucosal nodules <2 cm in diameter
  - Lymphomas: rare; account for <0.5% of all colorectal malignancies
  - Sarcomas: extremely rare; account for <0.1% of all large bowel malignancies
  - Symptoms and signs include abdominal pain, abdominal distention, obstipation, constipation

- **Differential Diagnosis**
  - Adenocarcinoma
  - Stricture: inflammatory or radiation-induced
  - Appendicitis
  - Diverticular disease

- **Treatment**
  - Lymphoma: for localized, low-grade colorectal lesions, radiation is usually first-line therapy; for intermediate- and high-grade lymphomas, chemotherapy combined with radiation therapy should be primary treatment
  - Sarcoma: radical en bloc excision to obtain a margin of uninvolved normal tissue
  - Carcinoid: surgery is mainstay of therapy; degree of resection depends on size (lesions >2 cm may require formal resection; lesions <2 cm may be amenable to local excision)
  - Prognosis: size is an extremely important prognostic factor; for sarcoma, significant prognostic indicators are tumor grade and size

- **Pearl**

Most rectal carcinoid tumors are limited in size and risk.

Reference

Soga J: Carcinoids of the colon and ileocecal region: A statistical evaluation of 373 cases collected from the literature. J Exp Clin Cancer Res 1998;17:139.

Colovesical Fistula

- ■ Essentials of Diagnosis
  - Fistula is a communication between 2 epithelialized surfaces, usually between bladder and GI tract
  - Causes include prior abdominal operation, especially for inflammatory bowel disease; malignancy; abscesses; diverticular disease; radiation; diverticulitis is most common cause
  - Symptoms and signs include chronic refractory urinary tract infection, fecaluria, pneumaturia
  - CT may detect small amounts of air in bladder; CT can locate the fistula and possible source (eg, sigmoid diverticulitis, mass, abscess)

- ■ Differential Diagnosis
  - Consider etiology of fistula formation and reasons for failed closure
  - These causes may include foreign body, radiation injury, abscess, distal obstruction, neoplasm, inflammatory conditions, epithelialization of the tract

- ■ Treatment
  - Up to 50% of colovesical fistulas from diverticulitis close spontaneously
  - Institute early, aggressive treatment of sepsis; drain abscesses; give IV antibiotics for infection
  - Surgery indications: recurrent urinary tract infection, failure of fistula to close spontaneously
  - Prognosis: mortality rate for all fistulas is 5–20%; sepsis is major determinant of mortality and morbidity from fistulas

- ■ Pearl

Allow inflammation to resolve before any attempt at operative correction.

Reference

Vasilevsky CA et al: Fistulas complicating diverticulitis. Int J Colorectal Dis 1998;13:57.

Diverticulitis

- ■ **Essentials of Diagnosis**
    - • Results from perforation or infection of colonic diverticulum; most common in sigmoid colon; becomes clinically significant when infection spreads through wall of colon into pericolic tissue; may lead to intra-abdominal abscess, peritonitis; may be complicated by colonic fistulas (colovesical, coloenteric)
    - • Symptoms and signs: patients may present with localized abdominal pain, constipation or increased frequency of defecation, fever, abdominal distention, pelvic or lower quadrant mass
    - • CT (with oral and IV contrast) shows effacement of pericolonic fat, abscess, bowel wall thickening

- ■ **Differential Diagnosis**
    - • Colonic or visceral malignancy
    - • Appendicitis
    - • Renal colic
    - • Other causes of bowel obstruction: stricture, incarcerated hernia, internal hernia
    - • Crohn disease
    - • Ulcerative colitis, ischemic colitis, antibiotic-associated colitis

- ■ **Treatment**
    - • Mild to moderate cases may be treated as outpatient with oral antibiotics; NPO, IV hydration, and IV broad-spectrum antibiotics for more serious cases
    - • Percutaneous catheter drainage if abscess found on CT and accessible
    - • Emergency surgery is required for free perforation, peritonitis; urgent surgery is needed for failure of medical therapy; elective surgery reserved for recurrent disease, fistulas

- ■ **Pearl**

Let acute inflammation resolve before operation if possible.

References

Baevsky R: Acute diverticulitis. N Engl J Med 1998;339:1082.
NIH Patient Information: http://digestive.niddk.nih.gov/ddiseases/pubs/diverticulosis/
Roberts P et al: Practice parameters for sigmoid diverticulitis. The Standards Task Force, American Society of Colon and Rectal Surgeons. Dis Colon Rectum 1995;38:125.

Diverticulosis

- **Essentials of Diagnosis**
  - Diverticulosis is the presence of multiple false diverticula; colonic diverticula are acquired and are classified as false because they consist of mucosa and submucosa that have herniated through the muscular coats
  - Diverticula are more common in the colon than in any other portion of the GI tract; 95% are in the sigmoid colon
  - Symptoms and signs: diverticulosis is asymptomatic in about 80% of people and is detected incidentally on barium enema x-rays or endoscopy, if it is discovered at all; patients may present with lower GI bleeding

- **Differential Diagnosis**
  - Diverticulitis
  - Neoplasm (colonic or anal)
  - Arteriovenous malformation

- **Treatment**
  - Asymptomatic persons with diverticulosis may be given a high-fiber diet
  - Surgery is indicated for massive hemorrhage or to rule out carcinoma in some patients
  - Prognosis: natural history of diverticulosis has not been defined; 10–20% of patients develop diverticulitis or hemorrhage when monitored for many years; 76% of complications of diverticular disease develop in patients with no prior colonic symptoms

- **Pearl**

Asymptomatic disease generally does not require treatment.

Reference

Young-Fadok TM et al: Colonic diverticular disease. Curr Probl Surg 2003;37:457.

Ogilvie Syndrome

- ■ Essentials of Diagnosis
  - • Massive colonic distention in the absence of mechanical obstruction; severe form of ileus; diagnosis of exclusion
  - • Risk factors include bedridden, elderly patients; orthopedic injuries; psychotropic medications or narcotics; metabolic disorders including hypothyroidism, diabetes, renal failure; collagen vascular diseases including lupus, amyloidosis, scleroderma
  - • Symptoms and signs include abdominal distention, without pain or tenderness initially; tympanitic abdomen to percussion
  - • Abdominal x-ray shows marked gaseous distention of colon, especially right colon; contrast enema confirms absence of mechanical obstruction

- ■ Differential Diagnosis
  - • Rule out mechanical obstruction

- ■ Treatment
  - • Nasogastric decompression and aggressive enema regimen provide resolution in 86% of patients
  - • Bowel rest
  - • Correct metabolic abnormalities
  - • Discontinue antimotility medications
  - • Colonoscopic decompression if cecum dilated >9–10 cm
  - • Surgery indications: failure to reduce dilation despite conservative measures and endoscopic intervention
  - • Medications: neostigmine (anticholinesterase) may help decompress colon (administration must be monitored)

- ■ Pearl

Ogilvie syndrome usually resolves with time and correction of electrolytes.

Reference

Paran H et al: Treatment of acute colonic pseudo-obstruction with neostigmine. J Am Coll Surg 2000;190:315.

Peutz-Jeghers Syndrome

- **Essentials of Diagnosis**
    - Multiple GI non-neoplastic hamartomas; polyps occur primarily in jejunum and ileum; can act as lead point for intussusception due to obstruction; predisposition to cancers
    - Familial autosomal dominant syndrome mapped to chromosome 19p13.3, which encodes serine/threonine kinase
    - Laboratory findings: hamartomas consist of supportive framework of smooth muscle tissue covered by hyperplastic epithelium

- **Differential Diagnosis**
    - Neoplasms of small bowel: adenocarcinoma, carcinoid tumor, leiomyoma/leiomyosarcoma

- **Treatment**
    - Remove polyps surgically; use endoscopic techniques when possible
    - Monitor treatment with screening for gonadal tumors and breast cancer

- **Pearl**

Carriers have an increased risk of cancers of the breast, testis, ovary, and gastrointestinal tract.

Reference

Bond JH: Polyp guideline: Diagnosis, treatment, and surveillance for patients with colorectal polyps. Practice Parameters Committee of the American College of Gastroenterology. Am J Gastroenterol 2000;95:3053.

Polyposis Syndromes

- ■ Essentials of Diagnosis
  - Familial adenomatous polyposis (FAP) (adenomatous polyposis coli) is a rare but important disease because colorectal cancer develops before age 40 in nearly all untreated patients
  - FAP is autosomal dominant disease; APC gene localized to chromosome 5q21
  - Extracolonic manifestations of FAP: endocrine adenoma, osteoma, epidermoid cyst, small bowel adenoma, visceral malignancy, desmoid tumor, thyroid carcinoma, hepatoblastoma
  - Gardner syndrome: variant of FAP with polyposis, desmoid tumors, osteomas of mandible or skull, and sebaceous cysts
  - Turcot syndrome: variant of FAP with polyposis and medulloblastoma or glioma
  - Symptoms and signs: most patients are asymptomatic
  - Lower endoscopy reveals numerous colonic or rectal polyps

- ■ Differential Diagnosis
  - Sporadic polyps
  - Sporadic colorectal adenocarcinoma

- ■ Treatment
  - Colectomy should be done
  - Indications for surgery: FAP has 100% penetrance for colorectal carcinoma
  - Abdominal colectomy (subtotal colectomy) with ileorectal anastomosis leaves risk of rectal carcinoma
  - Total colectomy and ileoanal pouch procedure are preferred for most patients, especially if numerous adenomas in the rectum
  - Prevention: when FAP is known in a family, relatives at risk should undergo annual surveillance endoscopy, beginning in their middle teens
  - Prognosis: desmoid tumors grow slowly and capriciously but are fatal in 10% of patients with FAP

- ■ Pearl

Always refer inherited cancer syndrome patients to genetic counseling for personal and family evaluation, documentation, and follow-up.

Reference

Calland JF et al: Genetic syndromes and genetic tests in colorectal cancer. Semin Gastrointest Dis 2000;11:207.

Polyps, Colorectal

- **Essentials of Diagnosis**
  - Colorectal polyps are masses of tissue that project into the lumen; types include neoplastic (adenomas, carcinomas), hamartomas, inflammatory, and hyperplastic
  - Prevalence of colonic and rectal adenomas is 30% at age 50 years, 40% at age 60, 50% at age 70, and 55% at age 80; 25% of patients who have 5 or more adenomatous polyps have a synchronous colon cancer at initial colonoscopy
  - Symptoms and signs: most polyps are asymptomatic, but the larger the lesion, the more likely it is to cause symptoms
  - Barium enema shows rounded filling defect with smooth, sharply defined margins; colonoscopy most reliable diagnosis with biopsy

- **Differential Diagnosis**
  - Malignant neoplasm
  - Artifacts seen on barium enema (eg, fecal matter, air bubbles, appendices epiploicae, lymph nodes) may be confused with polyps
  - Diverticula

- **Treatment**
  - Polyps of the colon and rectum are treated with polypectomy because they produce symptoms, they may be malignant when first discovered, or they may become malignant later
  - Surgery indications: large, sessile, soft, velvety lesions in the rectum are usually villous adenomas; these tumors have high malignant potential and must be excised completely
  - Consider open or laparoscopic colonic resection if colonoscopy is unsuccessful, lesion is large and sessile, or many polyps
  - Patients with HNPCC or multiple polyps may require total abdominal colectomy with ileorectal anastomosis
  - Prognosis: cancer is found in 1% of adenomas <1 cm in diameter, 10% of adenomas 1–2 cm in size, and up to 45% of adenomas >2 cm

- **Pearl**

  Consider a polyposis syndrome when there are multiple lesions.

References

Bond JH: Polyp guideline: Diagnosis, treatment and surveillance for patients with colorectal polyps. Practice Parameters Committee of the American College of Gastroenterology. Am J Gastroenterol 2000;95:3053.

NIH Patient Information: http://digestive.niddk.nih.gov/ddiseases/pubs/colonpolyps_ez/

Proctitis & Anusitis, Infectious

- **Essentials of Diagnosis**
  - Proctitis and anusitis are nonspecific terms for varying degrees of inflammation due to infectious or inflammatory diseases; causative agent or event determines symptoms, signs, and appropriate management
  - Herpes proctitis: lesions appear as vesicles, which rupture to form ulcers; ulcers may become secondarily infected; viral culture of vesicle or biopsy of ulcer is diagnostic
  - Anorectal syphilis: chancre is an indurated, nontender perianal ulcer at the site of inoculation; dark-field microscopy of exudate and serologic testing are preferred for diagnosis
  - Gonococcal proctitis: caused by the gram-negative diplococcus *Neisseria gonorrhoeae*; culture on Thayer-Martin medium reveals gram-negative diplococci; enzyme-linked immunosorbent and DNA probe assays are available
  - Chlamydial proctitis and lymphogranuloma venereum: causative agent is *Chlamydia trachomatis*; diagnosis is made with the lymphogranuloma venereum complement fixation test; tissue cultures are also used
  - Chancroid: *Haemophilus ducreyi* causes soft ulcer and local lymphadenitis; *H ducreyi* culture on heated blood agar supplemented with factor X is diagnostic

- **Differential Diagnosis**
  - Radiation-induced or ischemic proctitis

- **Treatment**
  - Herpes proctitis: oral acyclovir is the treatment of choice but is not curative
  - Anorectal syphilis: penicillin is treatment of choice
  - Gonococcal proctitis: intramuscular procaine penicillin G and oral probenecid
  - Chlamydial proctitis and lymphogranuloma venereum: tetracycline for 21 days
  - Chancroid from *H ducreyi:* azithromycin, erythromycin, ciprofloxacin, or ceftriaxone
  - Prevention: sexual contacts must be sought, tested, and treated

- **Pearl**

Always identify sexual contacts of patients with sexually transmitted diseases.

Reference

Rompalo AM: Diagnosis and treatment of sexually acquired proctitis and proctocolitis: An update. Clin Infect Dis 1999;28(suppl 1):S84.

Proctitis, Inflammatory & Radiation

- ■ Essentials of Diagnosis
  - • Inflammatory proctitis: a mild form of ulcerative colitis that is limited to the rectum; disease is often self-limited
  - • Radiation proctitis: due to radiation of the rectum; disease may develop months to years after the injury
  - • Symptoms and signs include rectal bleeding, discharge, diarrhea, and tenesmus; patients with late disease present with recurrent urinary tract infections, vaginal discharge, fecal incontinence, rectal bleeding, changes in stool caliber, constipation

- ■ Differential Diagnosis
  - • Infectious proctitis
  - • Crohn disease
  - • Malignancy

- ■ Treatment
  - • Inflammatory proctitis: corticosteroid retention enemas for 2 weeks; if no response, a short course of oral corticosteroids may be given
  - • Radiation proctitis: initial therapy includes bulk-forming agents, antidiarrheal and antispasmodic agents
  - • Treat late complications of radiation injury with dilatation of strictures and laser coagulation of telangiectasias; surgical success in treating fistulas to the bladder or vagina involves interposition or transposition of healthy nonirradiated tissue into the field; infrequently is the rectum so badly damaged that it must be removed

- ■ Pearl

Allow acute inflammation to resolve before any operative intervention.

Reference

Babb RR: Radiation proctitis: A review. Am J Gastroenterol 1996;91:1309.

Pruritus Ani

- ■ Essentials of Diagnosis
  - Severe perianal itching, often at night; when condition is chronic, skin becomes white, leathery, and thickened
  - Cause is usually idiopathic; pinworms (*Enterobius vermicularis*) are the most common cause of perianal itching in children

- ■ Differential Diagnosis
  - Other perianal lesions that distort normal anal anatomy, such as hemorrhoids, fistulas, fissures, tumors of the anorectum, previous surgery, and radiation therapy
  - Primary dermatologic diseases such as lichen planus, atopic eczema, psoriasis; contact dermatitis from local anesthetic creams or soaps
  - Perianal neoplasms such as Bowen disease and extramammary Paget disease

- ■ Treatment
  - Treat identifiable causes of pruritus ani (infection, hemorrhoids, contact dermatitis)
  - Prevention: educate patients to maintain proper perineal hygiene, avoid soaps and topical ointments, and keep perineum dry

- ■ Pearl

Keep area clean and dry.

Reference

Welton ML: Anorectum. In Way LW, Doherty GM (editors): Current Surgical Diagnosis & Treatment, 11th ed. McGraw-Hill, 2003.

Volvulus

- ■ Essentials of Diagnosis
  - Rotation of a segment of intestine on an axis (bowel twists on its mesentery); most commonly sigmoid colon (65%) and cecum; may produce large or small bowel obstruction
  - Symptoms and signs include severe, intermittent, colicky abdominal pain; abdominal distention; nausea, vomiting; constipation leading to obstipation
  - Abdominal x-ray shows "bent inner tube," signs of intestinal obstruction, including air-fluid levels and dilated loops of bowel
  - Perform abdominal x-ray, barium enema

- ■ Differential Diagnosis
  - Functional bowel obstruction: adynamic ileus, pseudo-obstruction
  - Other causes of mechanical obstruction: neoplasm, stricture, extrinsic compression, hernia (external or internal), adhesions

- ■ Treatment
  - Endoscopic evaluation and attempt at decompression for sigmoid volvulus
  - Placement of rectal tube
  - Exploratory laparotomy, untwisting of the bowel, and resection of ischemic or necrotic bowel
  - Surgery is indicated for peritoneal findings of strangulation or perforation, failure to resolve volvulus with endoscopic decompression, recurrence even after successful detorsion
  - Prognosis: mortality rate is 12% after emergent operation for cecal volvulus, 35% if cecum is gangrenous, and 50% for perforated sigmoid volvulus

- ■ Pearl

Rigid sigmoidoscopy can untwist nearly all sigmoid volvulus.

Reference

Chang GJ et al: Large intestine. In Way LW, Doherty GM (editors): Current Surgical Diagnosis & Treatment, 11th ed. McGraw-Hill, 2003.

22

Anorectum

Anal Canal Cancer

- ■ Essentials of Diagnosis
  - Tumors found anatomically from upper to lower border of internal anal sphincter, 6–12 mm above dentate line
  - Risk factors include: homosexual males; chronic anal infection (human papillomavirus [HPV]); history of anogenital warts; sexually transmitted disease; >10 sexual partners; cervical, vulvar, or vaginal cancer
  - Symptoms and signs include perianal irritation, usually long-standing; palpable mass, possibly indurated; bleeding; itching; tenesmus
  - Computed tomography and magnetic resonance imaging reveal anal mass; endorectal ultrasound reveals size and depth of invasion and perianal nodes
  - Workup: perform physical examination with digital rectal exam; assess for lymphadenopathy (groin); examination under anesthesia, anoscopy with biopsy; endorectal ultrasound

- ■ Differential Diagnosis
  - Tumor of anal margin, anal melanoma, low rectal cancer
  - Perianal or perirectal abscess or fistula
  - Hemorrhoids

- ■ Treatment
  - Chemoradiation is mainstay of therapy
  - Surgery is indicated for local excision of small, well-differentiated, mobile lesions confined to the submucosa; surgery is largely used as salvage procedure for recurrent or persistent disease (abdominoperineal resection)
  - Radiation therapy: 30 Gy to primary tumor and pelvic and inguinal nodes; mitomycin given on day 1 of radiation; two 4-day infusions of 5-fluorouracil on days 1 and 28 of chemoradiation therapy; cisplatin may be used in place of mitomycin
  - Prognosis: mobile lesions <2 cm have cure rates of 80%; tumors >5 cm have 50% mortality; 40% of patients die of disease outside pelvis; T1–T3 node-negative disease has 5-year survival of 88%; T1–T3 node positive has 5-year survival of 52%

- ■ Pearl

Always contact sexual partners of patients with sexually transmitted diseases.

References

Allal AS et al: Effectiveness of surgical salvage therapy for patients with locally uncontrolled anal carcinoma after sphincter-conserving treatment. Cancer 1999;86:405.

National Comprehensive Cancer Network: Practice Guidelines. http://www.nccn.org

Anal Fissure & Ulcer

- ■ Essentials of Diagnosis
  - Fissure: split in the anoderm; ulcer: chronic fissure, associated with skin tag (sentinel pile) once matured
  - Located in midline, distal to dentate line; most commonly posteriorly (90%); caused by forceful dilatation of anal canal, usually from defecation, leading to sphincter spasm and local anoderm ischemia
  - Symptoms and signs include pain and bleeding with defecation; pain may be tearing or burning, worst during defecation, may last for hours; constipation may develop from fear of recurrent pain
  - Physical examination reveals disruption of anoderm in midline at mucocutaneous junction; sentinel skin tag or pile may be present at inferior margin

- ■ Differential Diagnosis
  - Crohn disease
  - Anal tuberculosis
  - Anal malignancy
  - Abscess
  - Fistula
  - Cytomegalovirus

- ■ Treatment
  - Initial treatment is conservative with stool softeners, bulking agents, sitz baths
  - Surgery is indicated for failure of conservative measures; perform lateral internal anal sphincterotomy
  - Medications: 0.2% nitroglycerin ointment
  - Botulinum toxin infiltration into internal sphincters may aid healing
  - Prognosis: conservative measures achieve healing in 90% of cases; second episode has 70% chance of healing with conservative treatment; lateral internal anal sphincterotomy is >90% successful

- ■ Pearl

Bulking agents and softeners will heal most fissures.

Reference

Brisinda G et al: A comparison of injections of botulinum toxin and topical nitroglycerin ointment for the treatment of chronic anal fissure. N Engl J Med 1999;341:65.

Anal Margin Cancer

■ Essentials of Diagnosis

- Located at or outside the anal verge; usually well-differentiated, keratinizing tumors; behave similarly to squamous cell carcinomas of skin; 4 types: squamous cell, basal cell, Bowen disease, Paget disease
- Symptoms and signs include mass, bleeding, pain, discharge; basal cell: raised edges with central ulcer; Bowen disease: scaly, erythematous, sometimes pigmented; Paget disease: erythematous, eczematoid rash; often associated with condylomas in younger patients
- Endorectal ultrasound reveals size and depth of invasion and perianal nodes
- Workup: perform physical examination with digital rectal exam; assess for lymphadenopathy (groin); examination under anesthesia, anoscopy with biopsy; endorectal ultrasound

■ Differential Diagnosis

- Chronic or nonhealing perineal ulcer
- Anal canal cancer
- Perianal abscess
- Anal fissure

■ Treatment

- Small, well-differentiated lesions (<4 cm) may be treated with wide excision; large, deep lesions involving sphincters require abdominoperineal resection; grossly involved lymph nodes should be resected
- Bowen disease: wide local excision and 4-quadrant biopsy
- Paget disease: wide local excision; multiple perianal biopsies
- Prognosis: squamous cell carcinoma: T stage determines survival; 5-year survival for T1 100%, T2 60%; basal cell carcinoma: metastasis is rare; local recurrence is 30%; Bowen disease: invasive squamous cell carcinoma develops in <10%

■ Pearl

Mapping the extent of the process by multiple perianal biopsies will help to plan and monitor therapy.

References

Marchesa P et al: Perianal Bowen's disease: A clinicopathologic study of 47 patients. Dis Colon Rectum 1997;40:1286.

National Comprehensive Cancer Network: Practice Guidelines. http://www.nccn.org

Anorectal Abscess & Fistula

- **Essentials of Diagnosis**
  - Causes include occlusion of anal glands and crypts at the dentate line, impaction of vegetable matter or edema from trauma, inflammatory bowel disease (Crohn disease)
  - Abscesses are classified according to space they invade: supralevator, ischiorectal, superficial, intersphincteric, transsphincteric
  - Goodsall rule: used to identify direction of fistula tract; with anterior external opening, tract extends in a radial direction to the dentate line; with posterior external opening, fistula tract curves to the posterior midline
  - Symptoms and signs include severe anal or perianal pain, usually continuous and throbbing; severe, life-threatening perineal sepsis may develop; fistula has internal and external openings with mucopurulent drainage; fistulous tract is often palpable and firm
  - Imaging studies are unnecessary in uncomplicated cases; transrectal ultrasound may reveal extent of sphincter involvement

- **Differential Diagnosis**
  - Inflammatory bowel disease (Crohn disease)
  - Pilonidal disease
  - Hidradenitis suppurativa
  - Anal tuberculosis

- **Treatment**
  - Abscess: operative drainage
  - Intersphincteric abscess: internal sphincterotomy
  - Fistula-in-ano: fistulotomy, curettage of tract and granulation tissue, healing by secondary intention
  - Medications: antibiotics are not necessary unless patient is immunocompromised, diabetic, has extensive cellulitis, or has valvular heart disease
  - Prognosis: 50% of patients are cured with drainage alone

- **Pearl**

Drainage of a perirectal abscess can be successful without antibiotics; antibiotics cannot be successful without drainage.

Reference

Practice parameters for treatment of fistula-in-ano–supporting documentation. The Standards Practice Task Force. The American Society of Colon and Rectal Surgeons. Dis Colon Rectum 1996;39:1363.

Condylomata Acuminata

- ■ Essentials of Diagnosis
    - The most common sexually transmitted viral disease
    - Caused by HPV; multiple types have been identified: HPV-6 and HPV-11 are associated with common benign genital warts; HPV-16 and HPV-18 are associated with high-grade anal dysplasia and squamous cell anal cancer
    - Immunosuppression, either from drugs after transplantation or from human immunodeficiency virus, increases susceptibility to condylomatous disease, with prevalence rates of 5% and 85%, respectively
    - Symptoms and signs include pruritus, discharge, bleeding, odor, and anal pain; warts are isolated, clustered, or coalescent; warts tend to run in rows radiating out from the anus
    - Anoscopy and proctosigmoidoscopy are essential because disease extends internally in >75% of patients; condylomas should be biopsied to detect unsuspected low-grade or high-grade dysplasia or squamous cell carcinoma of the anal canal

- ■ Differential Diagnosis
    - Condylomata lata lesions of secondary syphilis
    - Anal squamous cell carcinoma

- ■ Treatment
    - Minimal disease is treated in the office with topical agents; more extensive disease may require initial treatment under anesthesia
    - Medications: topical agents include dichloroacetic acid or 25% podophyllum resin in tincture of benzoin
    - Patients should be seen at regular intervals until resolution is complete

- ■ Pearl

Always assess the anal canal for proximal disease, and always send biopsy tissue to assess for carcinoma.

Reference

Rompalo AM: Diagnosis and treatment of sexually acquired proctitis and proctocolitis: An update. Clin Infect Dis 1999;28(suppl 1):S84.

Hemorrhoids

- ■ Essentials of Diagnosis
  - • Internal hemorrhoids originate above dentate line, covered by mucosa; external hemorrhoids are vascular complexes covered by anoderm, below dentate line; no correlation between constipation and hemorrhoids
  - • Internal hemorrhoid classification: first-degree, bleeding; second-degree, bleeding and prolapse but spontaneously reduce; third-degree, bleeding, prolapse, and require manual reduction; fourth-degree, incarcerated
  - • External hemorrhoids become symptomatic with thrombosis
  - • Symptoms and signs: internal hemorrhoids cause bright red blood per rectum, mucus discharge, sense of rectal fullness, but no pain; may prolapse into the anal canal and may become strangulated and necrotic; external hemorrhoids cause sudden, severe perianal pain, itching; may be accompanied by a skin tag; thrombosed external hemorrhoids are a tense, tender subcutaneous mass with purple-black discoloration

- ■ Differential Diagnosis
  - • Anal fissure
  - • Anal ulcer
  - • Anorectal malignancy
  - • Inflammatory bowel disease

- ■ Treatment
  - • First- and most second-degree hemorrhoids: medical management initially, dietary alteration, addition of bulking agents, stool softeners, increased liquid intake, sitz baths
  - • Third- and fourth-degree lesions and incarcerated internal hemorrhoids: excisional hemorrhoidectomy; excise tissue and ligate vascular pedicle
  - • Surgery is indicated for failure of medical management; strangulated, thrombosed hemorrhoids
  - • Medications: stool softeners, bulking agents
  - • Lifestyle changes: increase fiber and exercise; decrease constipating foods; decrease time spent on commode and straining

- ■ Pearl
  Bulking agents and sitz baths can resolve dramatic-appearing hemorrhoids over several days without resection.

Reference
Komborozos VA et al: Rubber band ligation of symptomatic internal hemorrhoids: Results of 500 cases. Dig Surg 2000;17:71.

Rectal Fixation, Abnormal

- ■ Essentials of Diagnosis
  - • Attachment of the rectum to the sacrum has lengthened, allowing rectum to block defecation, protrude into the vagina, or prolapse through the anus; may be secondary to colonic dysmotility; female to male ratio is 5:1
  - • Symptoms and signs: internal intussusception causes rectal fullness, urge to defecate, mass; rectal prolapse causes bleeding, mucus discharge, tenesmus, incontinence, pain
  - • Histologic examination reveals diffuse submucosal cysts with a characteristic fibrotic pattern distinguishing them from colorectal malignancy
  - • Sigmoidoscopy may reveal circumferential intussusceptum or ulcerated mass that appears malignant; colonoscopy of entire colon is necessary to rule out malignancy
  - • Workup: patients with internal intussusception and rectal prolapse need anorectal manometry, pudendal nerve latency studies, defecography, and barium enema or colonoscopy

- ■ Differential Diagnosis
  - • Anorectal malignancy
  - • Prolapsed hemorrhoids

- ■ Treatment
  - • Mild to moderate intussusception: treat with bulking agents, modification of bowel habits, and reassurance
  - • Surgery for rectal prolapse: abdominal procedures are sigmoid resection with or without rectopexy and rectopexy alone; perineal operations consist of perineal rectosigmoidectomy and modified Delorme procedure
  - • Abdominal procedures achieve lower recurrence rate and preserve reservoir capacity of rectum but carry more risk; perineal procedures avoid intra-abdominal anastomosis but remove rectum, eliminate rectal reservoir, and have higher recurrence rates
  - • Abdominal procedures are preferred in low-risk, active patients <50 years and those who require other abdominal procedures
  - • Prognosis: addition of sigmoid resection at rectopexy lowers risks of recurrence and postoperative constipation without increasing morbidity

- ■ Pearl

Assess for other colon lesions before operation for prolapse.

Reference

Jacobs LK et al: The best operation for rectal prolapse. Surg Clin North Am 1997;77:49.

Rectal Ulcer, Solitary

- ■ Essentials of Diagnosis
  - Obliteration of rectal lamina propria by fibroblasts; may be clinically associated with and caused by pelvic floor abnormalities such as rectal prolapse, intussusception; results in defecation disorder with intense straining
  - Symptoms and signs include difficulty initiating bowel movements, possible rectal prolapse, fecal incontinence, sense of rectal fullness, tenesmus
  - On proctoscopy, most lesions are in anterior and anterolateral quadrants of rectal wall, 10–12 cm above anal verge; ulcers may be solitary, multiple, circumferential, usually shallow

- ■ Differential Diagnosis
  - Neoplasm
  - Stricture
  - Rectal prolapse
  - Rectal intussusception

- ■ Treatment
  - Treatment options range from dietary modification to biofeedback, rectopexy, coloanal anastomosis, diverting colostomy; therapy is based on severity of symptoms and associated diseases
  - Dietary modifications: increase daily fiber intake to 30–40 g; increase fluid intake; avoid caffeine and alcohol
  - Surgery is indicated for pelvic floor pathology (evident on defecography); rectal prolapse should be repaired with perineal proctectomy or rectopexy
  - Prognosis: the combination of dietary and bowel habit modifications provides reasonable relief in ~13%

- ■ Pearl

Biopsy suspicious lesions.

Reference

Welton ML: Anorectum. In Way LW, Doherty GM (editors): Current Surgical Diagnosis & Treatment, 11th ed. McGraw-Hill, 2003.

Rectovaginal Fistula

- **Essentials of Diagnosis**

  - Communication between anterior wall of the rectum and posterior wall of the vagina; tract is generally visible or palpable; causes passage of stool and flatus through the vagina
  - Causes include obstetric injury (most common), Crohn disease, diverticulitis, radiation, undrained cryptoglandular disease
  - Vaginogram or barium enema may identify the fistula; if fistula is not found on radiographic or physical examination, a dilute methylene blue enema may be administered with a tampon in vagina

- **Differential Diagnosis**

  - Obstetric injury
  - Crohn disease
  - Diverticulitis
  - Radiation
  - Undrained cryptoglandular disease

- **Treatment**

  - Inciting event (injury, inflammation, radiation) should be allowed to heal or subside before undertaking repair
  - About 50% of small rectovaginal fistulas secondary to obstetric trauma heal spontaneously
  - Fistulas due to cryptoglandular disease may close spontaneously once the primary process is drained
  - Fistulas secondary to Crohn disease rarely heal spontaneously
  - Fistulas due to radiation injury: if not amenable to local procedures, perform transabdominal resection and coloanal anastomosis
  - High rectovaginal fistulas: transabdominal approach allowing resection of diseased bowel involved in the fistula
  - Low, simple fistulas and some mid-rectovaginal fistulas: endorectal advancement of an anorectal flap

- **Pearl**

Always allow underlying inflammation to resolve to the greatest extent possible before operative repair of the fistula.

Reference

Hyman N: Endoanal advancement flap repair for complex anorectal fistula. Am J Surg 1999;178:337.

Section VII
Oncology & Endocrine Surgery

Chapters

23

Head & Neck

Head & Neck Squamous Cell Cancer

- ■ Essentials of Diagnosis
  - Tobacco and alcohol use account for 75% of oral, oropharyngeal, and hypopharyngeal cancers; second primary cancers develop in 10–15% of cases
  - Symptoms and signs include leukoplakia and erythroplakia as important premalignant lesions, pain (location correlates with tumor location), bleeding, obstruction, mass, otalgia, odynophagia, dysphagia, trismus, hoarseness
  - Computed tomography (CT) scan of the head and neck can show involvement of paranasal sinus and parapharyngeal and pterygomaxillary spaces, orbits, and anterior skull base; magnetic resonance imaging (MRI) of the head and neck can show cancer at the skull base, parapharyngeal space, and orbit
  - Workup: perform biopsy for definitive diagnosis (punch or fine-needle aspiration); examine under anesthesia (with direct laryngoscopy, nasopharyngoscopy, rigid esophagoscopy, and bronchoscopy)

- ■ Differential Diagnosis
  - Squamous cell carcinoma of the skin
  - Melanoma

- ■ Treatment
  - Multimodal: surgery, radiation therapy and chemotherapy, maxillofacial prosthetics, speech therapy
  - Prognosis: curable in 80% of cases when detected early
  - Prevention: discontinue tobacco and alcohol use

- ■ Pearl

Careful intraoral examination in smokers can reveal these lesions early.

References

Beenken SW et al: Work-up of a patient with a mass in the neck. Adv Surg 1996;28:371.

National Comprehensive Cancer Network: Practice Guidelines. http://www.nccn.org

Salivary Gland Infection

- **Essentials of Diagnosis**
  - Paired major salivary glands include parotid, submandibular, and sublingual glands; infectious and inflammatory diseases of the salivary glands are common and frequently involve the major glands, especially the parotids
  - Causes include actinomycosis, acute bacterial sialoadenitis, cat scratch disease, mumps, tuberculosis
  - Symptoms and signs include parapharyngeal edema; pain; fever; indurated, enlarged, tender gland; external pressure on the gland releases purulent material from gland opening
  - Workup: perform CT scan for suspected abscess, cultures of salivary secretions, possibly blood cultures (depending on degree of systemic illness)

- **Differential Diagnosis**
  - Salivary gland tumor
  - Lymphoma

- **Treatment**
  - Antibiotic therapy and fluid management are the mainstay of treatment of acute bacterial sialoadenitis
  - Surgery is indicated for lack of clinical improvement with antibiotics alone; aim of operation is to drain abscess

- **Pearl**

Lemon drops may help to stimulate salivary flow and drainage of infection.

Reference

Brook I: Acute bacterial suppurative parotitis: Microbiology and management. J Craniofac Surg 2003;14:37.

Salivary Gland Tumors

- ■ Essentials of Diagnosis
    - • Paired major salivary glands include parotid, submandibular, and sublingual glands; minor salivary glands are distributed in mucosa of the lips, cheeks, hard and soft palate, uvula, floor of mouth, tongue, and peritonsillar region
    - • Malignancy rates by gland: 15% of parotid tumors, 50% of submandibular tumors, 90% of minor salivary gland tumors; 70% of parotid tumors are pleomorphic adenomas (50% of all salivary gland tumors)
    - • Symptoms and signs include nodule in the parapharyngeal space, enlarged cervical lymph nodes, pain
    - • CT or MRI can identify extent of salivary gland mass, extension into surrounding nerves, and local nodal spread

- ■ Differential Diagnosis
    - • Benign neoplasms of the salivary gland: pleomorphic adenoma, mixed tumor, monomorphic adenoma, oncocytoma, Warthin tumor
    - • Malignant neoplasms of the salivary gland: acinic cell carcinoma, adenocarcinoma, adenoid cystic carcinoma, malignant mixed tumor, mucoepidermoid carcinoma, squamous cell carcinoma, undifferentiated carcinoma
    - • Rule out for swelling in the parotid gland: parotitis, enlarged preauricular or parotid lymph node, branchial cleft cyst

- ■ Treatment
    - • Benign tumors: remove surgically with margin of normal tissue
    - • Low-grade salivary gland cancers: complete excision is sufficient
    - • High-grade salivary gland cancers: usually require postoperative radiation therapy
    - • Clinically involved lymph nodes: remove by radical or modified radical neck dissection
    - • Prognosis: for stages I and II, 10-year survival is about 80%; for stages III and IV, 10-year survival is about 30%

- ■ Pearl

Most tumors in the superficial portion of the parotid gland can be removed by superficial parotidectomy.

References

National Comprehensive Cancer Network: Practice Guidelines. http://www.nccn.org
Spiro RH: Management of malignant tumors of the salivary glands. Oncology 1998;12:671.

Sialolithiasis

- ■ Essentials of Diagnosis
    - Both a cause and a consequence of chronic sialadenitis; 80–90% occur in the ducts of the submandibular glands; 20–40% of stones are radiolucent
    - Symptoms and signs include painful swelling; patients may complain of extrusion of gravel from the ducts; symptoms worsen with eating
    - CT scan may show sialoliths

- ■ Differential Diagnosis
    - Salivary tumors and infections
    - Lymphoma

- ■ Treatment
    - Intraoral removal of stones by ductal dilation and massage
    - Surgery for excision of the gland

- ■ Pearl

Lemon drops may help to stimulate salivary flow and drainage of infection.

Reference

Rowe LD: Otolaryngology–head & neck surgery. In Way LW, Doherty GM (editors): Current Surgical Diagnosis & Treatment, 11th ed. McGraw-Hill, 2003.

Sjögren Syndrome

■ Essentials of Diagnosis
- Chronic, systemic inflammatory disorder of unknown etiology; associated with rheumatoid disorders such as rheumatoid arthritis, scleroderma, and systemic lupus erythematosus
- Symptoms and signs include desiccated cornea and conjunctiva; 33% of patients have enlarged parotid glands; dry mouth, eyes, and other mucous membranes throughout the body
- Laboratory findings: Schirmer test measures quantity of tears secreted in 5 minutes in response to irritating stimuli; response is decreased in Sjögren syndrome; elevated levels of serum antibodies to gamma globulin, nuclear protein, and many tissue constituents; elevated rheumatoid factor (70% of cases); elevated erythrocyte sedimentation rate (70% of cases)

■ Differential Diagnosis
- Rule out lymphoma (44-fold increased risk in patients with Sjögren syndrome)

■ Treatment
- Artificial tears, saliva substitute
- Surgery (tarsorrhaphy) is indicated if artificial tears fail
- Oral corticosteroids or immunosuppressants are rarely indicated

■ Pearl

Evaluate for other autoimmune disease if Sjögren syndrome is suspected.

Reference

Belafsky PC, Postma GN: The laryngeal and esophageal manifestations of Sjögren's syndrome. Curr Rheumatol Rep 2003;5:297.

24

Thyroid & Parathyroid

Goiter, Simple or Nontoxic (Diffuse & Multinodular)

- ■ Essentials of Diagnosis
  - May be physiologic or pathophysiologic: physiologic occurs during puberty, menses, or pregnancy; pathophysiologic is due to iodine deficiency, congenital defect in thyroid hormone production, or goitrogenic foods or drugs; drugs implicated as goitrogens include lithium, p-aminosalicylic acid, aminoglutethimide, sulfonamides, phenylbutazone
  - Symptoms and signs include neck mass, inspiratory stridor, dyspnea, dysphagia
  - Ultrasound reveals size and extent of goiter and can define focal nodules; computed tomography (CT) and magnetic resonance imaging can define retrosternal or intrathoracic extension but are not primary diagnostic tools

- ■ Differential Diagnosis
  - Thyroid malignancy or lymphoma
  - Acute suppurative thyroiditis
  - Silent thyroiditis
  - Subacute thyroiditis
  - Reidel thyroiditis

- ■ Treatment
  - Multinodular goiter can be treated with operative removal, thyroid hormone administration, or radioactive iodine therapy; >90% of intrathoracic goiters can be removed through cervical incision
  - Surgery is indicated to relieve local compressive symptoms, to rule out cancer if suspicious areas of hardness or rapid growth occurs, and to resect proven malignancy
  - Medications: suppressive thyroxine (T_4), radioactive iodine 131 (^{131}I)

- ■ Pearl

Tracheal compression can make anesthesia induction the most dangerous part of the operation.

References

Mack E: Management of patients with substernal goiters. Surg Clin North Am 1995;75:377.

National Comprehensive Cancer Network: Practice Guidelines. http://www.nccn.org

Graves Disease

- **Essentials of Diagnosis**
  - Diffuse hypersecretory goiter causing increased levels of thyroid hormone in the blood; arises from stimulatory autoantibodies against thyroid-stimulating hormone (TSH) receptor
  - Symptoms and signs include nervousness, diaphoresis, heat intolerance, tachycardia, palpitations, fatigue, and weight loss; flushed and staring appearance; warm, thin, and moist skin; fine hair; exophthalmos
  - Laboratory findings show suppressed TSH; elevated triiodothyronine (T_3), free T_4, and radioactive iodine uptake; high thyroid-stimulating immunoglobulin level
  - Thyroid ultrasound reveals a diffusely enlarged gland, with or without nodules, and high vascular flow; diffuse increased uptake of radioiodine on radioiodine scan

- **Differential Diagnosis**
  - Anxiety neurosis
  - Pheochromocytoma
  - Primary ophthalmopathy (eg, orbital tumors)
  - Thyrotoxicosis factitia
  - Thyroiditis

- **Treatment**
  - Antithyroid drugs, radioactive iodine, or thyroidectomy
  - Surgery is indicated for very large goiter or multinodular goiter with relatively low radioactive iodine uptake, thyroid nodule that may be malignant, pregnant patients or children, women who wish to become pregnant within 1 year of treatment, patients who cannot maintain long-term follow-up
  - Medications: propylthiouracil, methimazole, radioiodine (^{131}I)

- **Pearl**

Most patients in the United States choose radioiodine as definitive therapy.

Reference

Ljunggren JG et al: Quality of life aspects and costs in treatment of Graves' hyperthyroidism with antithyroid drugs, surgery, or radioiodine: Results from a prospective randomized trial. Thyroid 1998;8:653.

Hashimoto Thyroiditis

- **Essentials of Diagnosis**
    - Autoimmune thyroiditis; may cause initial transient hyperthyroidism followed by chronic hypothyroidism
    - Symptoms and signs: dysphagia; initial inflammatory stage: enlarged, occasionally tender thyroid; chronic atrophic stage: shrunken, firm or nodular thyroid
    - Laboratory findings show elevated TSH, elevated titers of antimicrosomal and antithyroglobulin antibodies

- **Differential Diagnosis**
    - Associated with HLA-DR3, HLA-DR5, HLA-B8
    - Rule out thyroid lymphoma; thyroid carcinoma

- **Treatment**
    - Surgery is indicated for local symptoms of pressure, suspected malignancy, enlarging gland despite thyroid hormone replacement
    - Medications: thyroid hormone; occasionally, β-blocker is required initially to control symptoms of hyperthyroidism

- **Pearl**

Cancer is more frequent in patients with Hashimoto thyroiditis than in those without, so nodules must be evaluated carefully.

Reference

Singe PA: Thyroiditis: Acute, subacute and chronic. Med Clin North Am 1991;75:61.

Hürthle Cell Neoplasm

- **Essentials of Diagnosis**
  - More aggressive variant of follicular thyroid neoplasm; accounts for approximately 2% of all malignant thyroid tumors
  - Symptoms and signs include painless or enlarging thyroid nodule that is hard, rubbery, or soft; enlarged or hard cervical lymph nodes; hoarseness, dyspnea, stridor, dysphagia
  - Ultrasound shows solid or cystic nodule; nonfunctioning (cold) on radioiodine scan
  - Workup: measure serum TSH and calcium; perform fine-needle aspiration (FNA) biopsy

- **Differential Diagnosis**
  - FNA cannot reliably differentiate the atypical cells of invasive Hürthle adenocarcinoma from its counterpart benign adenoma
  - Hürthle cells are also frequently present on FNA of Hashimoto thyroiditis, but usually with accompanying lymphocytes
  - Rule out concurrent hyperparathyroidism

- **Treatment**
  - All Hürthle cell neoplasms should be excised unless Hürthle cell adenoma can be diagnosed with 100% certainty on FNA (not usual)
  - Medications: suppressive doses of thyroid hormone after thyroid ablation or thyroidectomy
  - Prognosis: worse outcome predicted by extensive angioinvasion, older age, presence of distant metastases

- **Pearl**

Hürthle cells on FNA are not necessarily a neoplasm; also look for evidence of Hashimoto thyroiditis.

References

Cooper D, Schneyer C: Follicular and Hürthle cell carcinoma of the thyroid. Endocrinol Metab Clin North Am 1990;19:577.

Dean DS, Hay ID: Prognostic indicators in differentiated thyroid carcinoma. Cancer Control 2000;7:229.

National Comprehensive Cancer Network: Practice Guidelines. http://www.nccn.org

Hypercalcemia of Malignancy, Humoral

- **Essentials of Diagnosis**
  - Hypercalcemia due to hormonal product of non-parathyroid cancer; most common cause of hypercalcemia in hospitalized patients
  - Laboratory findings show low intact parathyroid hormone (PTH) level, elevated PTH-related protein level, anemia, elevated serum calcium (sometimes >14 mg/dL), increased alkaline phosphatase activity

- **Differential Diagnosis**
  - Most common tumors causing ectopic hyperparathyroidism are squamous cell carcinoma of the lung, renal cell carcinoma, bladder cancer
  - Less common tumors are hepatoma; tumors of ovary, stomach, pancreas, parotid gland, or colon
  - Primary hyperparathyroidism

- **Treatment**
  - Treatment is directed at normalizing serum calcium
  - Effective treatment of primary tumor often improves malignancy-associated hypercalcemia
  - Medications: saline diuresis with furosemide; bisphosphonates, corticosteroids, gallium nitrate

- **Pearl**

Newer potent bisphosphonates protect the skeleton and maintain normal serum calcium levels.

References

National Comprehensive Cancer Network: Practice Guidelines. http://www.nccn.org

Ross JR et al: Systematic review of role of bisphosphonates on skeletal morbidity in metastatic cancer. BMJ 2003;327:469.

Strewler GJ, Nissenson RA: Hypercalcemia in malignancy. West J Med 1990;16:791.

Hypercalcemia, Familial Hypocalciuric

- **Essentials of Diagnosis**
    - Benign condition of chronic, nonprogressive hypercalcemia with mildly elevated intact PTH
    - Family history of hypercalcemia, especially in children
    - Caused by a defect in the gene coding for the calcium-sensing receptor; transmitted in an autosomal dominant fashion
    - Laboratory findings include high serum calcium, normal or mildly elevated intact PTH level, low urinary calcium, urinary calcium clearance to creatinine clearance ratio of <0.01, possibly high serum magnesium level

- **Differential Diagnosis**
    - Rule out primary hyperparathyroidism

- **Treatment**
    - None required
    - Operative neck exploration does not alleviate this condition (with the exception of total parathyroidectomy and surgically induced permanent hypoparathyroidism)
    - Genetic counseling is important; offspring homozygous for mutation have severe neonatal hyperparathyroidism, which is potentially lethal

- **Pearl**

Always consider familial hypocalciuric hypercalcemia in patients who have a calcium at or just above the upper limit of normal and PTH within 15% of the upper limit of normal.

Reference

Marx SJ et al: The hypocalciuric or benign variant of familial hypercalcemia: Clinical and biochemical features in fifteen kindreds. Medicine 1998;60:397.

Hyperparathyroidism, Primary

- ■ Essentials of Diagnosis
  - Excess secretion of PTH; most common cause of hypercalcemia in ambulatory patients; 83% are from single parathyroid adenoma, 6% multiple adenomas, 10% 4-gland hyperplasia, >1% parathyroid carcinoma
  - Symptoms and signs include fatigue, weakness, arthralgias, nausea, vomiting, dyspepsia, constipation, polydipsia, polyuria, nocturia, psychiatric disturbances, renal colic, bone and joint pain, nephrolithiasis and nephrocalcinosis, osteopenia, osteitis fibrosa cystica, peptic ulcer disease, gout, chondrocalcinosis, pancreatitis
  - Laboratory findings include elevated serum calcium, elevated intact PTH level, increased or normal urine calcium
  - Neck sestamibi scan may localize adenomatous parathyroid gland; neck ultrasound may localize abnormally large parathyroid gland

- ■ Differential Diagnosis
  - Primary hyperparathyroidism is part of the multiple endocrine neoplasia (MEN) syndromes, type 1 and 2A
  - Other causes of hypercalcemia include hyperthyroidism, Addison disease, pheochromocytoma, milk-alkali syndrome, vitamin D or A overdose, thiazides, familial hypocalciuric hypercalcemia, Paget disease

- ■ Treatment
  - Only successful treatment is parathyroidectomy; symptomatic and asymptomatic patients benefit from surgery (in terms of both symptoms and metabolism)
  - Treatment monitoring: immediately after surgery, oral calcium and possibly calcitriol will be needed for the short term
  - Prognosis: experienced surgeons have a success rate of 95% at initial surgery

- ■ Pearl

Intraoperative PTH monitoring has made directed parathyroidectomy an effective operative approach.

Reference

Clark OH: Changing surgical approaches to patients with primary hyperparathyroidism. Curr Surg 2000;57:546.

Hyperparathyroidism, Secondary

- **Essentials of Diagnosis**
  - Induced abnormality of endogenous mechanisms that ensure calcium homeostasis; increased PTH secretion in response to low plasma concentration of ionized calcium
  - Symptoms and signs include bone pain, pruritus, occasionally palpable parathyroid glands, skin changes if calciphylaxis present
  - Laboratory findings include elevated intact PTH level, low or normal serum calcium level, elevated serum phosphorous level (if due to renal disease), normal or low serum phosphorous level (if due to malabsorption or rickets)

- **Differential Diagnosis**
  - When associated with renal disease, often due to phosphate retention, failure of kidneys to generate 1,25 dihydroxyvitamin D, resistance of bones to PTH action, and decreased serum calcium concentration

- **Treatment**
  - Goal is to decrease stimulation of parathyroid gland by limiting serum hyperphosphatemia and supplementing both calcium and vitamin D; most cases manageable by medications and dialysis
  - Surgery: subtotal parathyroidectomy or total parathyroidectomy with parathyroid autograft; indications include hypercalcemia; normocalcemia with severe renal osteodystrophy or pruritus
  - Medications: oral or intravenous (IV) calcitriol; adjust calcium and phosphorous concentrations in dialysate solutions
  - Complications: profound hypocalcemia after subtotal parathyroidectomy for renal osteodystrophy because of "hungry bones" and decreased PTH secretion
  - Prognosis: 1–10% of patients with successful kidney grafting have persistent secondary hyperparathyroidism and hypercalcemia

- **Pearl**

A PTH level consistently >1000 pg/mL usually requires operative correction.

Reference

Tominaga Y: Surgical management of secondary hyperparathyroidism in uremia. Am J Med Sci 1999;317:390.

Hyperthyroidism, Non-Graves

- ■ Essentials of Diagnosis
  - Causes include solitary toxic adenoma, toxic multinodular goiter (Plummer disease), Jod-Basedow disease (thyrotoxicosis after iodine supplementation), amiodarone toxicity, TSH-secreting pituitary adenoma, human chorionic gonadotropin-secreting tumor (hydatidiform mole, choriocarcinoma), postpartum hyperthyroidism, struma ovarii (thyroid tissue in ovarian tumor, usually teratoma), factitious hyperthyroidism, iatrogenic hyperthyroidism
  - Symptoms and signs include nervousness, weight loss with increased appetite, heat intolerance, increased sweating
  - Laboratory findings include suppressed TSH (except in TSH-secreting pituitary adenoma); radioactive iodine uptake is generally 35–40% in toxic multinodular goiter

- ■ Differential Diagnosis
  - Jod-Basedow disease: iodine deficiency leads to a rise in TSH and thyroid growth; subsequent iodine supplementation can lead to thyrotoxicosis

- ■ Treatment
  - Multimodal, including antithyroid medication, radioactive iodine, or thyroid surgery
  - Percutaneous ethanol injections for solitary toxic adenoma have been used outside the United States (especially in Italy)
  - Surgery is indicated for large goiters causing compressive symptoms, suspicion of malignancy
  - Medications: propylthiouracil, methimazole, radioiodine (^{131}I)

- ■ Pearl

Hyperthyroidism with a nodule is one of the few remaining indications for thyroid scintiscan.

References

Fradkin JE, Wolff J: Iodide-induced thyrotoxicosis. Medicine 1983;62:1.
Jensen MD et al: Treatment of toxic multinodular goiter (Plummer's disease): Surgery or radioiodine? World J Surg 1986;10:673.

Hypoparathyroidism

- **Essentials of Diagnosis**
  - Uncommon condition usually occurs as a complication of thyroid surgery; can occur after any central neck resection (thyroid, parathyroid, or laryngeal)
  - Laboratory findings are hypocalcemia and hyperphosphatemia, low or absent urinary calcium, low or absent circulating PTH
  - Symptoms and signs include tetany, positive Chvostek sign (facial muscle twitch with tap over facial nerve) or Trousseau sign (forearm tetany with sphygmomanometer inflated), paresthesias, circumoral numbness, muscle cramps, irritability, carpopedal spasm, convulsions, opisthotonos, marked anxiety
  - Workup: make special note of previous neck surgery; perform serum and urine tests for calcium, phosphate, and PTH

- **Differential Diagnosis**
  - Rule out hypocalcemia from remineralization of bones after therapy for hyperparathyroidism
  - Pseudohypoparathyroidism (X-linked syndrome with defective renal adenylyl cyclase system)

- **Treatment**
  - Medications: oral calcium (calcium, lactate, or carbonate), calcitriol (0.25–1.0 µg/d), IV calcium gluconate for acute tetany (6 g mixed in 500 mL D5W, infused at 1 mL/kg/h)
  - Surgery: parathyroid autograft if cryopreserved; parathyroid allograft in hypoparathyroid patient with renal allograft
  - Prognosis: if postoperative hypocalcemia lasts longer than 2–3 weeks or if calcitriol therapy is required, hypoparathyroidism may be permanent

- **Pearl**

Prevention is far better than treatment; manage every parathyroid gland as if it is the last.

Reference

Lebowitz MR et al: Hypocalcemia. Semin Nephrol 1992;12:146.

Multiple Endocrine Neoplasia Type 1

- **Essentials of Diagnosis**
    - Also known as Wermer syndrome; characterized by tumors of the parathyroid, anterior pituitary, and pancreas; other tumors can include adrenocortical tumors, thymic or bronchial carcinoid tumors, multiple lipomas, cutaneous angiofibromas, and collagenomas; 90–97% of patients have biochemical evidence of hyperparathyroidism; 30–80% have pancreatic islet cell tumors; 15–50% develop pituitary tumors
    - Symptoms and signs: presentation depends on endocrine organ involved and the overproduction of specific hormone; symptoms may arise from pancreatic tumor mass itself
    - Laboratory findings include elevated serum calcium and intact PTH, elevated gastric acid secretion, elevated fasting serum gastrin level
    - Direct genetic testing generally offered only for probands with definitive evidence of MEN 1 syndrome; once the mutation is known, genetic testing of at-risk family members is useful
    - Workup: annual surveillance for adult gene carriers should include history and physical examination; calcium and PTH measurement for hyperparathyroidism; gastrin, pancreatic polypeptide, abdominal CT scan, and somatostatin receptor scintigraphy for pancreatic tumor detection; prolactin level for pituitary adenoma; chest CT scan for thymic carcinoid detection

- **Differential Diagnosis**
    - Hyperparathyroidism is due to multiple parathyroid adenomas with 4-gland involvement; main differential is the sporadic counterparts of the component diseases

- **Treatment**
    - Surgery is indicated for biochemical evidence of hyperparathyroidism or to remove or limit growth of pancreatic tumors (very often malignant)
    - Medications: H_2-receptor antagonists and proton pump inhibitors; bromocriptine to treat prolactinomas

- **Pearl**

Genetic counseling for family management is mandatory.

References

Brandi ML et al: Guidelines for diagnosis and therapy of MEN type 1 and type 2. J Clin Endocrinol Metab 2001;86:5658.

Doherty GM et al: Lethality of multiple endocrine neoplasia type 1. World J Surg 1998;22:581.

National Comprehensive Cancer Network: Practice Guidelines. http://www.nccn.org

Multiple Endocrine Neoplasia Type 2

- ■ Essentials of Diagnosis
  - • Group of syndromes caused by activating mutations of the *RET* proto-oncogene, including MEN 2A (Sipple syndrome), MEN 2B, familial medullary thyroid carcinoma
  - • MEN 2A: medullary thyroid carcinoma (MTC), pheochromocytomas, parathyroid hyperplasia
  - • MEN 2B: MTC, pheochromocytomas, mucosal neuromas, gangliomatosis of the gastrointestinal tract, distinctive marfanoid habitus
  - • Symptoms and signs include diarrhea, palpable thyroid nodule or multinodular thyroid gland, enlarged and firm cervical nodes (if metastatic disease)
  - • Laboratory findings include elevated calcitonin level if MTC has developed; elevated plasma metanephrines if pheochromocytoma
  - • Measure calcium and PTH; perform genetic screening for all patients with MTC

- ■ Differential Diagnosis
  - • MTC is usually the first abnormality in MEN 2A and 2B
  - • Pheochromocytomas are nearly always benign and limited to the adrenal medulla

- ■ Treatment
  - • Surgical resection is the only effective treatment for MTC
  - • Prophylactic operation for MTC based on direct genetic testing should be done before age 1 year for MEN 2B and age 5 years for most MEN 2A mutations
  - • Laparoscopic unilateral adrenalectomy for pheochromocytoma

- ■ Pearl

Genetic counseling for family management is mandatory.

References

Brandi ML et al: Guidelines for diagnosis and therapy of MEN type 1 and type 2. J Clin Endocrinol Metab 2001;86:5658.

National Comprehensive Cancer Network: Practice Guidelines. http://www.nccn.org

Osteitis Fibrosa Cystica

- Essentials of Diagnosis
  - End-stage skeletal manifestation of severe hyperparathyroidism; bone cysts, osteoporosis, and brown tumors (from excessive osteoclastic bone resorption)
  - Symptoms and signs include pain and pathologic fractures
  - Laboratory findings show elevated serum calcium, elevated intact PTH level
  - Radiographs show osteoporosis, fractures, cysts

- Differential Diagnosis
  - Rule out parathyroid carcinoma

- Treatment
  - The only effective treatment is localization and excision of all abnormal parathyroid tissue
  - Surgery (parathyroidectomy) is indicated for all patients
  - Medications: calcium and vitamin D supplementation postoperatively to aid in bone remineralization
  - Prognosis: reversal of bone loss is common after parathyroidectomy, but recovery of normal bone mass is rare

- Pearl

Intraoperative PTH monitoring has made directed parathyroidectomy an effective operative approach.

Reference

Agarwal G et al: Recovery pattern of patients with osteitis fibrosa cystica in primary hyperparathyroidism after successful parathyroidectomy. Surgery 2002;132:1075.

Paget Disease

- ■ Essentials of Diagnosis
    - Nonmalignant disease involving accelerated bone resorption followed by deposition of dense, disorganized, and ineffectively mineralized bone matrix
    - Three phases of disease: intense bone resorption; production of abundant woven bone with ineffective mineralization; deposition of sclerotic, chaotic cortical and trabecular bone
    - Symptoms and signs include pain in the affected bone
    - Laboratory findings include elevations of serum calcium, serum alkaline phosphatase, urine calcium, and urinary pyridinoline

- ■ Differential Diagnosis
    - Always consider metastatic disease to bone

- ■ Treatment
    - Treatment does not cure disease but prolongs remission; goals should include aggressive pain control
    - Medications: bisphosphonates to inhibit osteoclast resorption; injectable calcitonin
    - Monitor treatment with repeat radiographs, especially of weight-bearing joints, to detect degeneration

- ■ Pearl

Always consider metastatic disease to bone.

Reference

Schneider D et al: Diagnosis and treatment of Paget's disease of bone. Am Fam Physician 2002;65:2069.

Parathyroid Carcinoma

- ■ Essentials of Diagnosis
  - Affects 0.5–1% of patients with hyperparathyroidism; cancer is palpable in 50% of patients
  - Symptoms and signs include palpable neck mass, hoarseness, fatigue, depression, nausea, vomiting, dehydration, polydipsia, polyuria, pathologic fractures, nephrolithiasis (70% of patients)
  - Laboratory tests may show profound hypercalcemia, elevated intact PTH

- ■ Differential Diagnosis
  - Parathyroid carcinoma is suspected at operation if parathyroid is hard, whitish, has an irregular capsule, or is invasive; rarely diagnosed preoperatively
  - Differential diagnosis includes all causes of hypercalcemia

- ■ Treatment
  - Surgery: en bloc resection including ipsilateral thyroid lobe and central compartment lymph nodes; resection of local recurrent or metastatic disease if possible
  - Medications: palliative IV bisphosphonate to maintain eucalcemia; experimental immunization against PTH
  - Prognosis: with indolent malignancy, local and distant metastases occur over many years; 5-year survival rates are 40–69%

- ■ Pearl

A palpable neck mass in a patient with hyperparathyroidism is usually a thyroid nodule, but can be parathyroid cancer.

References

National Comprehensive Cancer Network: Practice Guidelines. http://www.nccn.org
Obara T, Fujimoto Y: Diagnosis and treatment of patients with parathyroid carcinoma: An update and review. World J Surg 1991;15:738.

Tertiary Hyperparathyroidism

- ■ Essentials of Diagnosis
  - Autonomous, hyperplastic parathyroid gland in a patient with secondary hyperparathyroidism; persistent hypercalcemia after normalization of renal function (usually with renal transplantation)
  - Laboratory findings include elevated intact PTH level, elevated serum calcium and phosphate levels

- ■ Differential Diagnosis
  - Primary hyperparathyroidism
  - Humoral hypercalcemia of malignancy

- ■ Treatment
  - Surgery is indicated for calcium-phosphate product >70, severe bone pain, pruritus
  - Medications: calcimimetics may have promise in the future
  - Prognosis: usually dramatic relief once symptoms are treated

- ■ Pearl

Intraoperative PTH monitoring has made directed parathyroidectomy an effective operative approach.

Reference

Pasieka JL et al: A prospective surgical outcome study assessing the impact of parathyroidectomy on symptoms in patients with secondary and tertiary hyperparathyroidism. Surgery 2000;128:531.

Thyroglossal Cyst

- ■ Essentials of Diagnosis
    - • Abnormal migration of the thyroid anlage during development can lead to a lingual thyroid or appear as a mass anywhere in the neck midline; persistence of thyroglossal duct leaves an epithelium-lined tract and can form a cyst that communicates with the foramen cecum at base of the tongue; tract of a persistent thyroglossal duct extends through the hyoid bone
    - • Symptoms and signs include a midline mass in the neck, which may be tender or asymptomatic

- ■ Differential Diagnosis
    - • Dermoid cyst
    - • Enlarged lymph nodes (especially Delphian)
    - • Thyroid cancer in pyramidal lobe

- ■ Treatment
    - • Lingual or ectopic thyroid should be excised
    - • Acute thyroglossal tract infections should be treated with heat, antibiotics, and incision and drainage (if indicated); complete tract excision (en bloc with middle of hyoid bone; Sistrunk procedure) once inflammation has subsided

- ■ Pearl

Thyroglossal duct abnormalities are midline; branchial cleft abnormalities are lateral.

Reference

Roback SA, Telander RL: Thyroglossal duct cysts and branchial cleft anomalies. Semin Pediatr Surg 1994;3:142.

Thyroid Cancer, Anaplastic

- **Essentials of Diagnosis**
  - Invasive, nonencapsulated tumor; represents 1% of all thyroid cancers; usually occurs later in life; 30% of patients have distant metastases at presentation
  - Symptoms and signs include firm or hard, fixed thyroid nodule or irregular anterior neck mass; quickly enlarging mass; may be tender; cervical lymphadenopathy; dyspnea or stridor; dysphagia or odynophagia

- **Differential Diagnosis**
  - Reliably diagnosed by FNA biopsy
  - Differential includes all other thyroid masses

- **Treatment**
  - Complete surgical resection is the best chance for cure, although local recurrence after surgical treatment is the rule
  - Combination chemotherapy and external-beam radiation offer the best palliation, but rarely curative
  - Tracheostomy below the tumor may be helpful for patients with actual or impending airway compromise
  - Prognosis: almost all patients die of local recurrence, pulmonary metastases, or both; life expectancy after diagnosis is typically 6 months; 1-year survival is 5–15%

- **Pearl**

Resection is useful for palliation if possible, but usually is not curative.

References

National Comprehensive Cancer Network: Practice Guidelines. http://www.nccn.org
Ordonez NG et al: Anaplastic thyroid carcinoma. Am J Clin Pathol 1991;96:15.

Thyroid Cancer, Follicular

- **Essentials of Diagnosis**
  - 10% of all malignant thyroid tumors; differentiated tumor develops from follicular cells; slightly worse prognosis than papillary thyroid cancer
  - Symptoms and signs include thyroid nodule that is hard, rubbery, or soft; enlarged or hard cervical lymph nodes; pain in the thyroid or paralaryngeal area; hoarseness; dyspnea; stridor; dysphagia
  - Ultrasound shows solid or cystic nodule; radioiodine scans show nonfunctioning (cold) nodule, usually not helpful; FNA biopsy is mainstay of evaluation

- **Differential Diagnosis**
  - FNA cannot reliably differentiate the atypical cells of invasive follicular adenocarcinoma from its counterpart benign adenoma
  - Follicular carcinoma is distinguished from follicular adenoma by capsular and vascular invasion on histologic studies

- **Treatment**
  - Surgery is indicated to remove all follicular thyroid cancers
  - External-beam radiation may palliate unresectable metastases resistant to radioiodine
  - Medications: suppressive doses of thyroid hormone after thyroid ablation or thyroidectomy; radioactive iodine therapy for remnant ablation or recurrent or metastatic disease
  - Prognosis: worse outcome predicted by extensive angioinvasion, older age, and distant metastases; 10-year survival nearly 100% with only microinvasion; 10-year survival about 72% with angioinvasion

- **Pearl**

  Older patients often present with distant metastasis.

References

Kebebew E et al: Differentiated thyroid cancer: "Complete" rational approach. World J Surg 2000;24:942.

National Comprehensive Cancer Network: Practice Guidelines. http://www.nccn.org

Thyroid Cancer, Medullary

- **Essentials of Diagnosis**
  - Aggressive, tenacious form of thyroid cancer that can be either sporadic or familial; 35% of MTC is familial
  - Symptoms and signs include hard thyroid nodule, enlarged or hard cervical lymph nodes, pain in the thyroid or paralaryngeal area, hoarseness, dyspnea
  - Laboratory tests show elevated calcitonin level (basal or calcium/pentagastrin stimulated)
  - Ultrasound demonstrates extent of tumor and can detect enlarged lymph nodes; no radioiodine uptake
  - Screen for *RET* mutations; 10% of patients without a family history have de novo mutations

- **Differential Diagnosis**
  - Tumors contain amyloid
  - Rule out MEN 2A or 2B

- **Treatment**
  - Prophylactic total thyroidectomy before age 5 years (MEN 2A) or 1 year (MEN 2B) recommended for patients without symptoms and with positive family genetic screening
  - Surgery is indicated for all MTCs, with central neck dissection; lateral neck dissection depends on size of tumor
  - Monitor treatment with calcitonin level and neck palpation every 3–6 months
  - Prognosis: 10-year survival is 30–40%

- **Pearl**

Always do direct genetic testing for RET proto-oncogene abnormality in patients with MTC.

References

Chi DD, Moley JF: Medullary thyroid carcinoma. Genetic advances, treatment recommendations, and the approach to the patient with persistent hypercalcitoninemia. Surg Oncol Clin North Am 1998;7:681.

National Comprehensive Cancer Network: Practice Guidelines. http://www.nccn.org

Thyroid Cancer, Papillary

- ■ Essentials of Diagnosis
  - • History of radiation to the neck in some patients
  - • Symptoms and signs include solitary thyroid nodule, enlarged or hard cervical lymph nodes, pain in the thyroid or paralaryngeal neck, hoarseness, dyspnea, stridor, dysphagia
  - • Ultrasound shows solid or cystic nodule; radioiodine scan shows nonfunctioning (cold) nodule
  - • Workup: measure serum TSH and calcium levels; perform FNA biopsy

- ■ Differential Diagnosis
  - • Grows slowly and metastasizes through lymph nodes; growth may be stimulated by TSH
  - • Differential includes all other thyroid masses

- ■ Treatment
  - • All papillary thyroid cancers should be excised, as well as bulky or palpable nodal recurrences
  - • Medications: suppressive doses of thyroid hormone after thyroid ablation or thyroidectomy; radioactive iodine therapy for remnant ablation and recurrent or metastatic disease
  - • Prognosis: very good even with metastases; 10-year survival after operation for papillary cancer is >80%

- ■ Pearl

Stage depends on age for differentiated thyroid cancer.

References

Kebebew E et al: Differentiated thyroid cancer: "Complete" rational approach. World J Surg 2000;24:942.

National Comprehensive Cancer Network: Practice Guidelines. http://www.nccn.org

Thyroid Lymphoma

- **Essentials of Diagnosis**
  - Often a history of hypothyroidism, specifically Hashimoto thyroiditis; median age at onset is the late seventh decade
  - Symptoms and signs include rapidly enlarging neck mass, hoarseness, stridor, dysphagia, odynophagia; thyroid is firm and fixed
  - Cancer staging: stage IE is disease within the thyroid gland; stage IIE is disease confined to the thyroid and regional lymph nodes; stage IIIE is disease on both sides of the diaphragm; stage IV is disseminated disease

- **Differential Diagnosis**
  - Anaplastic thyroid carcinoma
  - Other thyroid cancers

- **Treatment**
  - Little role for surgical therapy except incisional biopsy for diagnosis and lymphoma subtyping
  - Multiple-agent chemotherapy and radiation therapy are mainstays of treatment; radiation therapy can abrogate airway compromise

- **Pearl**

Excisional biopsy is often preferable to needle biopsy to determine lymphoma subtype.

Reference

National Comprehensive Cancer Network: Practice Guidelines. http://www.nccn.org

Thyroid Metastasis

- ■ Essentials of Diagnosis
  - Primary tumor types include renal, lung, breast, melanoma, head and neck tumors
  - FNA biopsy demonstrates metastatic carcinoma

- ■ Differential Diagnosis
  - Evaluate for primary thyroid tumors
  - If tumor is proved metastatic, identify primary and other sites of metastatic disease to make a comprehensive plan

- ■ Treatment
  - Surgery is indicated for inconclusive biopsy or occult primary tumor
  - Prognosis: outcome is poor; one series indicated that 11 of 12 patients died within 9 months of diagnosis

- ■ Pearl

Thyroidectomy for isolated metastasis is rarely a curative procedure.

References

Lin JD et al: Clinical and pathologic characteristics of secondary thyroid cancer. Thyroid 1998;2:149.

National Comprehensive Cancer Network: Practice Guidelines. http://www.nccn.org

Thyroid Nodule

■ Essentials of Diagnosis

- Very common (~5% of the population); central diagnostic question is whether the lesion is benign or malignant; only 5% of nodules represent thyroid cancer
- Laboratory tests include serum TSH level (low in solitary toxic nodule; normal or elevated in nonfunctioning nodules)
- FNA biopsy can have the following results: malignant, benign, indeterminate, inadequate; ultrasound can distinguish size and character (solid or cystic) of nodules and assess for nonpalpable nodules
- Workup: perform complete history and physical examination, focusing on duration of swelling, recent growth, local symptoms (dysphagia, pain, voice changes), and systemic symptoms (hyperthyroidism, hypothyroidism); the patient's age, sex, place of birth, family history, and history of head or neck irradiation are most important; perform thyroid function tests, thyroid ultrasound, FNA biopsy

■ Differential Diagnosis

- Rule out thyroid cancer

■ Treatment

- Surgery is indicated for obstruction of aerodigestive tract, FNA biopsy with malignant or indeterminate result, 3 successive inadequate biopsies, or recurrence of cyst after 2 aspirations
- Medications: TSH suppression with L-thyroxine if patient is hypothyroid; may arrest nodule growth

■ Pearl

Perform FNA only if the patient and physician are willing to monitor the nodule if the result is benign.

References

National Comprehensive Cancer Network: Practice Guidelines. http://www.nccn.org
Wong CK et al: Thyroid nodules: Rational management. World J Surg 2000;24:934.

Thyroiditis, Acute Suppurative

- ■ Essentials of Diagnosis
  - Sudden onset; often follows upper respiratory tract infection; peak incidence in childhood or young or middle-aged adults
  - Symptoms and signs include acute neck pain, exacerbated by neck extension; dysphagia; fever; chills; neck enlargement; warmth and erythema
  - Laboratory findings show leukocytosis, normal thyroid function
  - Thyroid ultrasound shows partially cystic mass
  - Perform guided needle aspiration, with Gram stain and culture of aspirate

- ■ Differential Diagnosis
  - Chronic suppurative thyroiditis
  - de Quervain thyroiditis

- ■ Treatment
  - Primary treatment is antibiotics
  - Thyroid abscess should be operatively drained
  - Prognosis: improvement should occur within 48–72 hours of starting antibiotics, with complete resolution after 2–4 weeks

- ■ Pearl

Most thyroid lesions are nontender; if tender, suspect infection.

Reference

Miyauchi A et al: Piriform sinus fistula: An underlying abnormality common in patients with autosuppurative thyroiditis. World J Surg 1990;14:400.

Thyroiditis, de Quervain, Subacute

- ■ Essentials of Diagnosis
  - • Noninfectious disorder; also known as subacute or giant cell thyroiditis; male to female ratio is 5:1
  - • Symptoms and signs include thyroid swelling, head and chest pain, weakness, fever, malaise, palpitations, weight loss, dysphagia, odynophagia
  - • Laboratory findings show elevated erythrocyte sedimentation rate, elevated serum gamma globulin, increased or normal thyroid hormone function tests
  - • Imaging shows decreased uptake on radioiodine thyroid scan

- ■ Differential Diagnosis
  - • Graves disease
  - • Thyroid cancer
  - • Acute suppurative thyroiditis

- ■ Treatment
  - • Illness is usually self-limited
  - • Medications: aspirin, ibuprofen, or corticosteroids relieve symptoms
  - • Prognosis: patients usually become euthyroid; 10% of patients have permanent hypothyroidism

- ■ Pearl

Always evaluate for carcinoma.

Reference

Singer PA: Thyroiditis: Acute, subacute and chronic. Med Clin North Am 1991;75:61.

Thyroiditis, Riedel

- **Essentials of Diagnosis**
  - Rare condition; invasive fibrosis of the thyroid gland; symptoms appear gradually
  - Symptoms and signs include large, nontender, woody mass in central neck; stridor; dysphagia; hoarseness
  - Laboratory findings include marked fibrosis and chronic inflammation on biopsy; hypothyroidism (late stage)

- **Differential Diagnosis**
  - Inflammatory process involves surrounding muscles and causes tracheal compression or esophageal obstruction
  - Rule out thyroid carcinoma; acute suppurative thyroiditis

- **Treatment**
  - Corticosteroids are first-line therapy; patient often requires long-term maintenance therapy
  - Low-dose radiation may be beneficial if corticosteroid therapy or resection is unsuccessful
  - Prognosis: multifocal fibrosis develops in some patients up to 10 years after diagnosis; condition may be life-threatening and can include retroperitoneal fibrosis

- **Pearl**

Always evaluate for thyroid carcinoma.

Reference

Girod DA et al: Riedel's thyroiditis: Report of a lethal case and review of the literature. Otolaryngol Head Neck Surg 1992;107:591.

25

Breast

Breast Cancer, Female

- ■ Essentials of Diagnosis
  - • Risk factors include higher education in women who have delayed childbearing, family history of breast cancer, personal history of breast cancer or some types of mammary dysplasia
  - • Distribution of cancers by quadrant: 45% in upper outer, 15% in upper inner, 5% in lower inner, 10% in lower outer, 25% in subareolar
  - • Symptoms and signs include palpable mass (90% detected first by patient); nipple discharge, especially bloody; nipple erosion; breast erythema or edema; skin or nipple retraction or dimpling; thickening in a portion of breast; adenopathy (axillary or supraclavicular)
  - • Imaging shows mammographic abnormality of increased density with microcalcifications and irregular border; ultrasound demonstrates solid mass (vs cyst, which is usually benign)
  - • Workup includes bilateral mammograms and tissue diagnosis

- ■ Differential Diagnosis
  - • Benign breast tumors
  - • Mastitis
  - • Fibrocystic disease

- ■ Treatment
  - • Surgery is indicated for stages I–III disease; options include lumpectomy, axillary interrogation, and postoperative radiation versus modified radical mastectomy
  - • Medications: adjuvant chemotherapy, hormonal therapy, or both for most patients with tumors >1 cm in diameter
  - • Prognosis: cancer localized to breast has 75–90% cure rate; with spread to axilla, 5-year survival is 40–50%, 10-year survival is 25%; positive factors include estrogen receptor expression and lack of her2/neu overexpression

- ■ Pearl

The rule of concordance for breast mass investigation: if a lesion is benign by examination, imaging, and cytology, then it can be followed up; otherwise, it should be excised.

References

Margolese RG: Surgical considerations for invasive breast cancer. Surg Clin North Am 1999;351:1451.

National Comprehensive Cancer Network: Practice Guidelines. http://www.nccn.org

Breast Cancer, Male

- ■ Essentials of Diagnosis
  - Painless lump beneath the areola in a man who is usually >50 years; nipple discharge, retraction, or ulceration may be present
  - Symptoms and signs may include gynecomastia and axillary or supraclavicular adenopathy
  - Mass is evident on mammography

- ■ Differential Diagnosis
  - Rule out gynecomastia; metastatic cancer from another site
  - Blood-borne metastases are often present at initial presentation, although may be latent

- ■ Treatment
  - Modified radical mastectomy is first-line therapy for surgical candidates; tumor hormone receptor status may help determine role of adjuvant chemotherapy
  - Prognosis: worse prognosis, stage for stage, than female breast carcinoma; respective 5- and 10-year survival rates are as follows: for stage I cancer, 58% and 38%; for stage II cancer, 38% and 10%; for all stages combined, 36% and 17%

- ■ Pearl

Carefully investigate the family history for an inherited tendency to disease.

References

Memon MA et al: Male breast cancer. Br J Surg 1997;84:433.
National Comprehensive Cancer Network: Practice Guidelines. http://www.nccn.org

Breast Lesions, Benign

- **Essentials of Diagnosis**
  - Types of lesions include mammary dysplasia (fibrocystic disease), fibroadenoma of the breast, intraductal papilloma, fat necrosis, mastitis, breast abscess
  - Fibrocystic disease: multiple painful bilateral masses, rapid fluctuation in mass size, symptoms increase during premenstrual phase of cycle
  - Fibroadenoma: round, firm, discrete, mobile mass
  - Intraductal papilloma: unilateral bloody nipple discharge
  - Fat necrosis: mass with associated skin or nipple retraction
  - Mastitis or breast abscess: area of erythema, tenderness, and induration
  - Ultrasound can distinguish solid from cystic mass; always perform mammography, ultrasound, or both; biopsy if any possibility of cancer

- **Differential Diagnosis**
  - Most common causative pathogen in mastitis and breast abscess is *Staphylococcus*
  - Rule out breast carcinoma

- **Treatment**
  - Nursing can continue with mastitis but should be discontinued with breast abscess; mastitis is treated with antibiotics that cover *Staphylococcus,* and drainage for abscess
  - Surgery is indicated for persistent dominant mass, mass after cyst aspiration, fibroadenoma (excisional biopsy), intraductal papilloma (total excision through circumareolar incision)
  - Prognosis is excellent

- **Pearl**

The rule of concordance for breast mass investigation: if a lesion is benign by examination, imaging, and cytology, then it can be followed up; otherwise, it should be excised.

Reference

Marchant DJ: Controversies in benign breast disease. Surg Oncol Clin North Am 1998;7:285.

Carcinoma, Inflammatory Breast

- Essentials of Diagnosis
  - Name refers to clinical appearance, not histologic subtype of mammary carcinoma; skin and subcutaneous tissue appear inflamed because of invasion of subdermal lymphatics by carcinoma
  - Symptoms and signs include breast mass; erythematous, edematous, warm skin on breast; failure to respond to antibiotics (if initially diagnosed as breast cellulitis) within 1–2 weeks; peau d'orange changes, most notable over dependent portions of the breast
  - Biopsy shows invasion of subdermal lymphatics

- Differential Diagnosis
  - Metastases tend to occur early and widely
  - Rule out mastitis or breast abscess

- Treatment
  - Multimodal treatment with external-beam radiation, chemotherapy, and hormonal therapy
  - Mastectomy is indicated for local control of disease
  - Medications: anthracycline-based combination chemotherapy
  - Prognosis: 5-year survival is about 50%

- Pearl

Always biopsy the inflamed-looking skin in patients with persistent apparent cellulitis.

References

Gradishar WJ: Inflammatory breast cancer: The evolution of multimodality treatment strategies. Semin Surg Oncol 1996;12:352.

National Comprehensive Cancer Network: Practice Guidelines. http://www.nccn.org

Gynecomastia

- ■ Essentials of Diagnosis
    - Hypertrophy of normal breast tissue; can be divided into 2 categories: pubertal hypertrophy (ages 13–17), senescent hypertrophy (age >50)
    - Associated with some recreational and therapeutic drugs: marijuana, digoxin, thiazides, estrogens, phenothiazines, theophylline
    - Symptoms and signs include unilateral or bilateral breast enlargement
    - Workup: biopsy dominant mass if concern for malignancy

- ■ Differential Diagnosis
    - Frequently no identifiable cause; may represent local manifestation of systemic illness such as hepatic or renal insufficiency or alterations in steroid metabolism
    - Rule out carcinoma of the breast

- ■ Treatment
    - Surgery is indicated if enlargement does not regress and breast is cosmetically unacceptable

- ■ Pearl

The rule of concordance for breast mass investigation: if a lesion is benign by examination, imaging, and cytology, then it can be followed up; otherwise, it should be excised.

Reference

Daniels IR, Layer GT: Gynaecomastia. Eur J Surg 2001;167:885.

Mondor Disease (Thrombophlebitis of the Thoracoepigastric Vein)

- **Essentials of Diagnosis**
  - Thrombophlebitis of the thoracoepigastric vein over breast or upper abdomen; more common in women; self-limited and often resolves within 3 weeks
  - Symptoms and signs include breast pain; superficial abdominal pain; localized tender, cordlike structure in subcutaneous tissue of abdomen, thorax, or axilla
  - Workup: perform physical examination; occasionally, soft-tissue ultrasound

- **Differential Diagnosis**
  - Rule out infectious process

- **Treatment**
  - Supportive symptomatic treatment with warm compresses
  - Medications: nonsteroidal anti-inflammatory drugs

- **Pearl**

Tenderness similar to that of fibrocystic disease but extending inferior to breast over costal margin often represents Mondor thrombophlebitis.

Reference

Bejanga BI: Mondor's disease: Analysis of 30 cases. J R Coll Surg Edinb 1992;37:322.

Paget Disease of Breast

- ■ Essentials of Diagnosis
  - Infiltrating ductal carcinoma involving the nipple epithelium; represents 1% of all breast cancers; 50–60% of patients have a palpable tumor
  - Symptoms and signs include burning and pruritus of the nipple, superficial erosion or ulceration of the nipple, serous or bloody nipple discharge, nipple retraction
  - Mammography may show thickening of the nipple, calcifications, or lesion anywhere in the breast
  - Workup: perform bilateral mammograms; biopsy the nipple erosion

- ■ Differential Diagnosis
  - Rule out inflammatory breast carcinoma

- ■ Treatment
  - Multimodality treatment is the same as for carcinoma of the female breast
  - Surgery indications: may consider excision of nipple-areola complex alone if no palpable tumor and no extensive disease visualized on mammogram; otherwise mastectomy
  - Prognosis: if no underlying mass and treated by modified radical mastectomy, 10-year survival is 82–100%

- ■ Pearl

Biopsy all persistent irritated lesions of the nipple.

Reference

Chaudry MA et al: Paget's disease of the nipple: A ten-year review including clinical, pathological, and immunohistochemical findings. Breast Cancer Res Treat 1986;8:139.

26

Adrenals

Adrenal Incidentaloma

■ Essentials of Diagnosis

- Found in 1–4% of computed tomography (CT) scans, 6% of random autopsies; incidence increases with age; >80% are nonfunctioning cortical adenomas; 5% each are preclinical Cushing syndrome, pheochromocytoma, and adrenocortical carcinoma; 2% are metastatic carcinoma
- Workup: all patients, even without hypertension, should have plasma metanephrines analyzed for pheochromocytoma and have overnight dexamethasone suppression test; hypertensive patients: measure serum potassium, plasma aldosterone, and renin activity; if tumor nonfunctional by hormone studies, size of tumor and patient's overall medical condition determine management; if metastasis is suspected and pheochromocytoma is ruled out, perform CT-guided fine-needle aspiration

■ Differential Diagnosis

- Simple adrenal cyst, myelolipoma, and adrenal hemorrhage can be identified by CT alone
- Adrenal mass >3 cm in a patient with previously treated malignancy is probably metastasis

■ Treatment

- Surgery is indicated for hormonally active tumor, tumor >4 cm, imaging not consistent with benign adenoma, increasing size on interval imaging
- Treatment monitoring: small, nonfunctioning tumors are almost always benign adenomas; follow with CT scan for size changes

■ Pearl

Biopsy adrenal tumor only if biochemical testing proves that it is not a pheochromocytoma and metastasis is suspected.

Reference

Young WF et al: Management approaches to adrenal incidentalomas: A review from Rochester, Minnesota. Endocrinol Metab Clin North Am 2000;29:159.

Adrenal Tumors, Sex Hormone–Producing

- ■ Essentials of Diagnosis
  - Two types, virilizing and feminizing; virilization is due to hypersecretion of adrenal androgens, mainly dehydroepiandrosterone (DHEA), its sulfate derivative (DHEAS), and androstenedione; estrogens are not normally synthesized by adrenal cortex
  - Symptoms and signs: virilization includes hirsutism, male-pattern baldness, acne, deep voice, male musculature, irregular menses, or amenorrhea; feminization occurs in men or causes precocious puberty in girls
  - Laboratory tests: virilizing adrenal tumors elevate DHEA, DHEAS, androstenedione, and testosterone; feminizing adrenal tumors elevate plasma or urine estrogens

- ■ Differential Diagnosis
  - Feminizing adrenal tumors are almost always malignant
  - Rule out congenital adrenal hyperplasia, ovarian tumors, testicular feminization, exogenous estrogen administration

- ■ Treatment
  - Surgery is indicated for all virilizing or feminizing adrenal tumors
  - Laparoscopic approach is reserved for tumors that do not appear malignant

- ■ Pearl

Feminizing tumors and tumors that cause multiple hormonal syndromes are almost always malignant.

References

Del Gaudio AD et al: Virilizing adrenocortical tumors in adult women. Cancer 1993;72:1997.

Goto T et al: Oestrogen producing adrenocortical adenoma: Clinical, biochemical, and immunohistochemical studies. Clin Endocrinol (Oxf) 1996;45:643.

National Comprehensive Cancer Network: Practice Guidelines. http://www.nccn.org

Adrenocortical Carcinoma

- ■ Essentials of Diagnosis
  - • Variety of clinical symptoms result from excess production of adrenal hormones
  - • Symptoms and signs are those of specific hormone excess (cortisol excess, virilization, feminization); also palpable abdominal mass, abdominal pain, fatigue, weight loss, fever, hematuria
  - • Magnetic resonance imaging (MRI) of adrenal glands: adrenocortical carcinomas are typically isodense relative to liver on T1-weighted MRI and hyperdense to liver on T2-weighted MRI; MRI more accurate than CT to gauge the extent of any intracaval tumor thrombus; perform detailed anatomic imaging of both adrenal glands (by CT or MRI) and potential sites of intra-abdominal metastasis (especially liver)
  - • Laboratory studies should always include plasma metanephrines to rule out medullary tumor (pheochromocytoma)

- ■ Differential Diagnosis
  - • Mean diameter of adrenal carcinoma at diagnosis is 12 cm
  - • Rule out pheochromocytoma

- ■ Treatment
  - • Laparoscopic surgery not recommended because of potential spread of tumor, fragility of tumor, and possible need to resect adjacent involved organs
  - • Medications: mitotane (an adrenolytic agent) can be used as adjuvant therapy; efficacy not proven
  - • Prognosis: recurrence is common despite an apparently complete resection; median survival is 25 months; 5-year actuarial survival is 25%; 5-year survival with grossly complete surgical resection is 50%

- ■ Pearl

The best opportunity to cure adrenal carcinoma is at an initial, radical operation.

References

National Comprehensive Cancer Network: Practice Guidelines. http://www.nccn.org
Stratakis CA et al: Adrenal cancer. Endocrinol Metab Clin North Am 2000;29:15.

Aldosteronoma (Primary Hyperaldosteronism)

- ■ Essentials of Diagnosis
  - Causes include aldosteronoma (75%) and bilateral adrenal hyperplasia (25%)
  - Symptoms and signs include hypertension, headaches, malaise, muscle weakness, polyuria, polydipsia, hypokalemic paralysis (rare)
  - Laboratory tests show hypokalemia, elevated aldosterone secretion, suppressed plasma renin activity, elevated aldosterone to renin ratio (>20; usually >30)
  - CT scan with thin sections through adrenals can identify most adenomas; perform laboratory evaluation including electrolytes, serum aldosterone, and renin levels; bilateral adrenal vein sampling for aldosterone if findings are equivocal

- ■ Differential Diagnosis
  - Rule out pheochromocytoma

- ■ Treatment
  - Surgery for patients with aldosteronoma and unilateral primary adrenal hyperplasia; these types of primary hyperaldosteronism are the most amenable to surgical correction; nearly always use a laparoscopic approach
  - Medications: spironolactone is a competitive aldosterone antagonist
  - Prognosis: removal of aldosteronoma normalizes potassium, but hypertension is not always cured

- ■ Pearl

Adrenal vein sampling can provide definitive lateralization of the problem in equivocal cases.

Reference

Ghose RP et al: Medical management of aldosterone-producing adenomas. Ann Intern Med 1993;153:2125.

Hyperadrenocorticism (Cushing Disease and Syndrome)

- ■ Essentials of Diagnosis
  - • Due to chronic glucocorticoid excess; includes Cushing disease (excess adrenocorticotropic hormone [ACTH] produced by pituitary adenomas) and Cushing syndrome (ectopic ACTH syndrome, or primary adrenal disease resulting in glucocorticoid secretion independent of ACTH stimulation)
  - • Symptoms and signs include truncal obesity, hirsutism, moon facies, acne, buffalo hump, purple striae, hypertension, hyperglycemia, weakness, depression, growth retardation or arrest in children
  - • Laboratory: overnight, low-dose dexamethasone suppression test and measurement of urinary free cortisol establish diagnosis; once Cushing syndrome established, measure plasma ACTH level: normal or elevated ACTH suggests pituitary adenoma or ectopic ACTH secretion; suppressed ACTH indicates hyperadrenocorticism due to primary adrenal disease
  - • Directed imaging includes pituitary MRI; abdominal CT or MRI

- ■ Differential Diagnosis
  - • Ectopic ACTH syndrome is usually caused by small-cell lung cancers or carcinoids

- ■ Treatment
  - • Resection is best treatment for cortisol-producing adrenal tumors or ACTH-producing tumors; includes transsphenoidal resection for pituitary adenoma; bilateral adrenalectomy for Cushing disease if pituitary surgery fails; unilateral adrenalectomy for unilateral adrenal adenomas or carcinomas
  - • Medications: ketoconazole, metyrapone, aminoglutethimide all control hypercortisolism by inhibiting steroid biosynthesis
  - • Prognosis: natural history of Cushing syndrome depends on underlying disease and varies from mild, indolent disease to rapid progression and death

- ■ Pearl

Recovery of the hypothalamic-pituitary-adrenal axis after resection of tumor causing adrenal-dependent Cushing syndrome takes 12–24 months.

Reference

Findling JW, Raff H: Newer diagnostic techniques and problems in Cushing's disease. Endocrinol Metab Clin North Am 1999;28:191.

Pheochromocytoma

- **Essentials of Diagnosis**
  - Found in <0.1% of patients with hypertension; associated with familial syndromes such as multiple endocrine neoplasia types 2A and 2B, Recklinghausen disease, von Hippel-Lindau disease; rule of 10s: 10% malignant, 10% familial, 10% bilateral, 10% multiple tumors, 10% extra-adrenal
  - Symptoms and signs include episodic or sustained hypertension; triad of palpitations, headache, and diaphoresis; anxiety; tremors; dizziness; nausea and vomiting
  - Laboratory findings show elevated plasma metanephrines; elevated 24-hour urine metanephrines
  - CT or MRI shows unilateral or bilateral lesions; metaiodobenzylguanidine (MIBG) scan shows asymmetric uptake (scan useful only for extra-adrenal, multiple, or malignant pheochromocytomas; not indicated for patients with biochemical diagnosis and unilateral lesion on cross-sectional imaging)

- **Differential Diagnosis**
  - Early recognition during pregnancy is essential because if pheochromocytoma is left untreated, half of fetuses and nearly half of mothers will die
  - Rule out other causes of hypertension, hyperthyroidism, anxiety disorder

- **Treatment**
  - α-Adrenergic blocking agents should be started once biochemical diagnosis is established to restore blood volume, prevent a severe crisis, and allow recovery from cardiomyopathy
  - Surgery is indicated for all pheochromocytomas
  - Medications: α-adrenergic blocking agents such as phenoxybenzamine (10–40 mg orally three times a day); β-adrenergic blocking agents only after full α-blockade achieved
  - Monitor treatment with plasma metanephrines after resection
  - Prognosis: treatment with ^{131}I-MIBG may help patients with metastatic or recurrent malignant pheochromocytomas

- **Pearl**

One presentation of pheochromocytoma is sudden death, underline sudden, underline death.

References

Duh QY: Evolving surgical management for patients with pheochromocytoma [editorial]. J Clin Endocrinol Metab 2001;86:1477.

Kebebew E et al: Benign and malignant pheochromocytoma: Diagnosis, treatment, and follow up. Surg Oncol Clin North Am 1998;7:765.

27

Sarcoma, Lymphoma, & Melanoma

Desmoid Tumor

- Essentials of Diagnosis
  - Soft-tissue neoplasm that originates from aponeurotic tissues; referred to as "aggressive fibromatosis" and behaves as low-grade malignant lesion; strongly associated with familial polyposis syndromes; increased frequency in patients with familial adenomatous polyposis, classically in the mesentery after total proctocolectomy
  - Symptoms and signs include enlarging, often painless, soft-tissue mass
  - Plain films may demonstrate visceral displacement or obstruction; abdominal pelvic computed tomography (CT) scan or magnetic resonance imaging (MRI) shows a soft-tissue mass; radiographically indistinguishable from soft-tissue sarcoma
  - Workup: perform radiography for tumor extent; core needle biopsy or incisional biopsy to establish diagnosis

- Differential Diagnosis
  - Soft-tissue sarcoma
  - Abdominal wall metastases

- Treatment
  - Mesenteric desmoids associated with familial adenomatous polyposis: manage conservatively for as long as possible
  - Surgery is indicated for resectable abdominal wall desmoid tumor; bowel obstruction secondary to desmoid that does not respond to conservative treatment
  - Medications: tamoxifen, sulindac; chemotherapy is last resort
  - Prognosis: tumors virtually never metastasize but are locally invasive, so location of tumor predicts prognosis

- Pearl

Although benign, the local effects of desmoid can be very destructive to surrounding normal tissues.

References

National Comprehensive Cancer Network: Practice Guidelines. http://www.nccn.org
Soravia C et al: Desmoid disease in patients with familial adenomatous polyposis. Dis Colon Rectum 2000;43:363.

Gastrointestinal Stromal Tumors, Leiomyomas, & Leiomyosarcomas

- **Essentials of Diagnosis**
  - Represent 1% of gastrointestinal (GI) malignancies; stomach is most common site; difficult to distinguish malignant from benign histologically; tumors may grow into gastric lumen, remain entirely on serosal surface, or become pedunculated within abdominal cavity
  - Symptoms and signs: often asymptomatic; may present with occult or apparent GI bleeding (melena, hematochezia), weight loss
  - Endoscopy usually shows a central ulceration on tumor; CT provides useful information on extragastric extension
  - Workup: endoscopic biopsy, perhaps guided by endoscopic ultrasound, is usually diagnostic

- **Differential Diagnosis**
  - Adenocarcinoma
  - Lymphoma
  - Other gastric neoplasms

- **Treatment**
  - Leiomyomas: enucleation or wedge resection (2–3 cm margin)
  - Leiomyosarcomas: more radical gastric resection
  - Medications: imatinib mesylate
  - Prognosis: GI stromal tumor has 5-year survival rate of 20–55% after resection

- **Pearl**

The availability of an effective systemic agent (imatinib mesylate) has revolutionized therapy of GI stromal tumor.

References

DeMatteo RP et al: Two hundred gastrointestinal stromal tumors: Recurrence patterns and prognostic factors for survival. Ann Surg 2000;231:51.

National Comprehensive Cancer Network: Practice Guidelines. http://www.nccn.org

Hodgkin Lymphoma

- **Essentials of Diagnosis**
  - Malignant neoplasm that originates in lymphoid tissue; characterized by Reed-Sternberg cells; several histologic subtypes based on lymphocyte infiltration: nodular sclerosis, 70%; mixed cellularity, 20%; lymphocyte predominance, 6%; lymphocyte depletion, 2%
  - Symptoms and signs: constitutional symptoms that lead to a "B" designation include fever, drenching night sweats, weight loss
  - Workup: perform excisional biopsy of enlarged lymph node; bone marrow biopsy; CT scans of neck, chest, abdomen, and pelvis

- **Differential Diagnosis**
  - Reactive lymphadenopathy
  - Metastatic disease to the lymph nodes

- **Treatment**
  - Surgery: excisional lymph node biopsy to establish diagnosis
  - Medications: the 2 common chemotherapy regimens are MOPP (mechlorethamine, vincristine, procarbazine, prednisone) and ABVD (doxorubicin, bleomycin, vinblastine, dacarbazine)
  - Prognosis: cure rate is >70%

- **Pearl**

Excisional biopsy is often preferable to needle biopsy to determine lymphoma subtype.

References

Advani RH, Horning SJ: Treatment of early-stage Hodgkin's disease. Semin Hematol 1999;36:270.

National Comprehensive Cancer Network: Practice Guidelines. http://www.nccn.org

Lipoma

- ■ Essentials of Diagnosis
  - Slow-growing, benign adipose tumor, most often in subcutaneous tissues; also may occur in deeper tissues such as intramuscular septa, thoracic cavity, abdominal organs, GI tract
  - Symptoms and signs include nontender, oval, mobile subcutaneous mass; deep lipoma typically presents as nontender and nonmobile soft-tissue mass
  - MRI may be able to differentiate between lipoma and liposarcoma; also useful for deep lesions or when malignancy is suspected

- ■ Differential Diagnosis
  - Fibroma
  - Epidermoid cyst
  - Desmoid tumor
  - Soft-tissue sarcoma (especially liposarcoma)

- ■ Treatment
  - Surgical excision of symptomatic or enlarging lesions
  - Lesions not easily encompassed by a subsequent re-excision (eg, >4 cm initially, or in sensitive areas around joints or on face) should be assessed initially by incisional biopsy to confirm benign histology before complete excision

- ■ Pearl

Multiple lipomas occur in some families, often with many subcutaneous, slightly tender angiolipomas; also present in multiple endocrine neoplasia type 1.

References

Jablons D et al: Thoracic wall, pleura, mediastinum, & lung. In Way LW, Doherty GM (editors): Current Surgical Diagnosis & Treatment, 11th ed. McGraw-Hill, 2003.
National Comprehensive Cancer Network: Practice Guidelines. http://www.nccn.org

Melanoma

- **Essentials of Diagnosis**

    - Four histologic categories of melanoma: superficial spreading (70%), nodular melanoma (15%), lentigo maligna melanoma (4–10%), acral lentiginous melanoma (2–8%)
    - Symptoms and signs: lesions suspicious for melanoma may be identifiable by A-B-C-D: asymmetry, border irregularity, color (variable or dark pigmentation), diameter (>6 mm)
    - CT or MRI can detect metastatic disease or evaluate noncutaneous melanomas; positron emission tomography may demonstrate areas of metastatic disease not detected with conventional CT or MRI
    - Workup: perform excisional biopsy (1- to 2-mm margins) or punch biopsy of the suspicious lesion

- **Differential Diagnosis**

    - Dysplastic nevi
    - Benign mole
    - Nonmelanotic skin cancer

- **Treatment**

    - Wide local excision: <1 mm thick, 1-cm margin; 2–4 mm thick, 2-cm margin; >4 mm thick, ≥2-cm margin
    - Sentinel lymph node biopsy for lesions >0.75 mm thick or thinner lesions with high-risk pathology (eg, ulcerated, many mitoses)
    - Adjuvant immunotherapy in patients with lymph node involvement or metastatic disease; radiation therapy to lymph node basins for patients with >10 positive lymph nodes
    - Medications: adjuvant interferon-α2b improves disease-free and overall survival for deep primary (IIB) or node-positive disease (III)
    - Prognosis: most important factors are vertical height of melanoma, sentinel lymph node status, number of positive lymph nodes, presence of metastatic disease

- **Pearl**

    Evaluate suspicious skin lesions with A-B-C-D: asymmetry, border irregularity, color (variable or dark pigmentation), diameter (>6 mm).

References

Balch CM et al: Efficacy of 2-cm surgical margins for intermediate-thickness melanomas (1 to 4 mm). Results of a multi-institutional randomized surgical trial. Ann Surg 1993;218:262.

National Comprehensive Cancer Network: Practice Guidelines. http://www.nccn.org

Non-Hodgkin Lymphoma

- **Essentials of Diagnosis**
  - Wide spectrum of lymphoid-derived tumors; may originate from B cells, T cells, or histiocytes; functionally separated into low grade and high grade
  - Symptoms and signs include nontender enlargement of lymph nodes, fever, drenching night sweats, weight loss
  - Workup: perform excisional biopsy of enlarged lymph node; bone marrow biopsy; CT scans of neck, chest, abdomen, and pelvis

- **Differential Diagnosis**
  - Reactive lymphadenopathy
  - Metastatic disease to the lymph nodes
  - Hodgkin disease

- **Treatment**
  - Treatment depends on grade and stage of lymphoma
  - Low-grade localized: radiation with or without adjuvant chemotherapy
  - Low-grade systemic: "watch and wait" approach; when more aggressive disease develops, single-agent palliative chemotherapy
  - High-grade localized: radiation and adjuvant chemotherapy
  - High-grade systemic: chemotherapy with or without radiation (to areas of bulky disease)
  - Medications: chemotherapy is classically the CHOP regimen (cyclophosphamide, doxorubicin, vincristine, prednisone) for high-grade systemic disease and extranodal lymphomas
  - Prognosis: depends on grade and type of malignancy; although low-grade lymphomas are typically indolent, they are difficult to cure and most patients eventually die of disease; median survival is 6–12 years; high-grade lymphomas have high rate of early disease-related mortality but are often curable with aggressive chemotherapy regimens

- **Pearl**

Excisional biopsy is often preferable to needle biopsy to determine lymphoma subtype.

References

Mounter PJ, Lennard AL: Management of non-Hodgkin's lymphomas. Postgrad Med J 1999;75:2.

National Comprehensive Cancer Network: Practice Guidelines. http://www.nccn.org

Retroperitoneal Sarcoma

- ■ Essentials of Diagnosis
  - Represents 15% of all sarcomas and 55% of all retroperitoneal tumors; most common variant is liposarcoma; metastasizes via hematogenous route, typically to liver or lung
  - Symptoms and signs typically include nonspecific, vague abdominal symptoms; early satiety; weight loss
  - Chest film or thoracic CT scan demonstrates pulmonary metastases; abdominal CT scan or MRI shows soft-tissue neoplasm and its relationship to adjacent retroperitoneal structures
  - Workup: perform abdominal pelvic CT scan or MRI (preferred) to evaluate extent of lesion; image-guided core needle biopsy; open or laparoscopic incisional biopsy; biopsy often best performed at beginning of definitive resection for diagnostic confirmation

- ■ Differential Diagnosis
  - Retroperitoneal lesions: teratoma, cyst, abscess, hematoma
  - Adrenal mass
  - Renal cell carcinoma

- ■ Treatment
  - Neoadjuvant chemoradiation often used to try to shrink tumor
  - Complete surgical extirpation with en bloc resection of involved structures
  - Operative excision in all patients with no evidence of metastases and if all gross tumor can be removed (~50% of cases)
  - Resection of pulmonary metastases considered in patients who have achieved local control and who have <4 pulmonary lesions; no definitive evidence to support adjuvant therapy
  - Prognosis: worse than for trunk or extremity sarcomas; most patients eventually die of disease, often with local recurrence

- ■ Pearl

Prognosis is largely dependent on grade of disease.

References

Moley JF, Eberlein TJ: Soft-tissue sarcomas. Surg Clin North Am 2000;80:687.
National Comprehensive Cancer Network: Practice Guidelines. http://www.nccn.org

Soft-Tissue Sarcoma

- **Essentials of Diagnosis**
  - 50% of masses arise in lower extremities, most commonly the thigh, others in retroperitoneum; originate from a wide variety of mesenchymal cell types and include liposarcoma, fibrosarcoma, rhabdomyosarcoma, leiomyosarcoma, desmoid tumors; sarcomas generally metastasize via hematogenous route, typically to lung
  - Familial syndromes that genetically predispose to soft-tissue sarcomas: Gardner syndrome (desmoid tumors), Recklinghausen disease (neurofibrosarcomas), Li-Fraumeni syndrome
  - Symptoms and signs: asymptomatic, large soft-tissue mass
  - MRI defines the extent of sarcoma and invasion of surrounding structures
  - Workup: core needle biopsy or incisional biopsy for histologic diagnosis; radiography to define extent of tumor and invasion of surrounding structures; evaluate for pulmonary metastases

- **Differential Diagnosis**
  - Traumatic injury
  - Hematoma
  - Cutaneous neoplasm or metastasis
  - Abscess

- **Treatment**
  - Wide local excision with a 2-cm margin; postoperative radiation for all high-grade sarcomas and those >2 cm
  - Resection of pulmonary metastases in patients who have achieved local control and have <4 lesions
  - Prognosis: >50% will eventually die of disease

- **Pearl**

Diagnostic biopsy must be planned to allow inclusion of tract within incisions at planned definitive resection.

References

Brennan MF et al: The role of multimodality therapy in soft-tissue sarcoma. Ann Surg 1991;214:328.
Moley JF, Eberlein TJ: Soft-tissue sarcomas. Surg Clin North Am 2000;80:687.
National Comprehensive Cancer Network: Practice Guidelines. http://www.nccn.org

Section VIII
Pediatric Surgery

Biliary Atresia

- ### Essentials of Diagnosis
  - Presents within first few weeks of life; 67% of patients ultimately require liver transplantation
  - Symptoms and signs include progressive jaundice in newborns 2–4 weeks old, mild hepatomegaly, failure to feed well, growth failure
  - Laboratory findings show hyperbilirubinemia
  - Imaging: technetium 99m–iminodiacetic acid (Tc-IDA) scan shows normal uptake into liver but failure to empty through bile duct into duodenum; ultrasound shows small or absent gallbladder, absence of choledochocele
  - Workup: perform liver function tests, α_1-antitrypsin level, Tc-IDA scan, ultrasound

- ### Differential Diagnosis
  - Biliary hypoplasia or Alagille syndrome
  - Other causes of neonatal jaundice
  - α_1-Antitrypsin deficiency

- ### Treatment
  - Portoenterostomy (Kasai operation) when proximal bile ducts of adequate caliber are located (150 μm in diameter ideal); liver transplantation if >1 year of age and liver failure or growth retardation occurs after portoenterostomy
  - Prognosis: 66–75% have bile flow after portoenterostomy if done before 60 days of age; bile flow unlikely if portoenterostomy performed after 120 days of life

- ### Pearl

Liver transplantation offers the best opportunity for a positive long-term outcome.

Reference

Narkowicz MR: Biliary atresia: An update on our understanding of this disorder. Curr Opin Pediatr 2001;13:435.

Cystic Disease of Lungs, Congenital

■ Essentials of Diagnosis

- Uncommon aberrations of respiratory tract development; often present early in life; some remain occult until adulthood
- Tracheobronchial atresia: can occur at any level; diffuse disease is fatal
- Isolated bronchial atresia: bronchus with blind pouch leads to compression of surrounding lung and emphysematous changes
- Bronchogenic cysts: can result from abnormal budding of foregut; usually single, lined by cuboidal respiratory epithelium, found in lower lobes; may communicate with tracheobronchial tree; can enlarge rapidly and rupture, causing tension pneumothorax
- Bronchopulmonary dysplasia: cluster of diseases including pulmonary agenesis, aplasia, primary and secondary hypoplasia
- Pulmonary sequestration: abnormal budding of foregut leading to lung parenchyma without bronchial communication
- Cystic adenomatoid malformation: overgrowth of terminal bronchiolar structures lined by respiratory epithelium with disorganized elastic connective tissue and smooth muscle
- Congenital lobar emphysema: hypoplastic bronchial cartilage in 25–75% of patients
- Workup: perform chest film, esophagography; chest computed tomography (CT) to exclude other diagnoses

■ Differential Diagnosis

- Any congenital cystic lesion of the lung
- Tumor
- Pneumonia

■ Treatment

- Tracheobronchial atresia: emergency tracheostomy is life-saving for isolated subglottic atresia
- Bronchogenic cysts: simple or segmental resection, rarely lobectomy
- Bronchopulmonary dysplasia (pulmonary aplasia): resect pulmonary stump
- Pulmonary sequestration: segmental resection or lobectomy
- Cystic adenomatoid malformation: surgical resection may be required in neonates with acute respiratory distress
- Congenital lobar emphysema: lobectomy

■ Pearl

Always consider congenital abnormality in adults with unusual pulmonary density.

Reference

Eber E, Zach MS: Long term sequelae of bronchopulmonary dysplasia (chronic lung disease of infancy). Thorax 2001;56:317.

Cystic Fibrosis

■ Essentials of Diagnosis

- Autosomal recessive disorder; defect in chloride transport results in excess NaCl absorption in the airway; airway secretions are low in volume and high in viscosity
- Symptoms and signs include recurrent respiratory infection, fever, chest pain
- Laboratory finding: positive sweat test (NaCl in sweat)

■ Differential Diagnosis

- Bronchogenic carcinoma
- Bronchiectasis
- Abscess
- Bacterial pneumonia

■ Treatment

- Double lung transplantation is indicated for end-stage pulmonary disease
- Complications include chronic bronchitis obliterans, a major obstacle and the cause of eventual transplant failure
- Prognosis: 1-year survival after transplantation is 85%; 5-year survival is 50%

■ Pearl

Consider this diagnosis in a child with chronic pulmonary symptoms.

Reference

Fiel SB: Clinical management of pulmonary disease in cystic fibrosis. Lancet 1993;341:1070.

Diaphragmatic Hernia, Congenital

- **Essentials of Diagnosis**
  - Occurs in 1/5000 to 1/2000 births; 80% are left-sided and 20% are right-sided
  - Symptoms and signs include dyspnea, chest retractions, decreased breath sounds on affected side
  - Prenatal ultrasound is accurate in 40–90% of cases, showing herniation of abdominal contents in thorax
  - Workup: obtain chest film, arterial blood gas measurements, echocardiogram; ultrasound for neural tube defects

- **Differential Diagnosis**
  - Associated neural tube defects
  - Associated cardiac defects

- **Treatment**
  - Primary repair or mesh repair once respiratory status has been optimized
  - Prognosis: 39–95% survival
  - Prevention: intrauterine repair is under investigation

- **Pearl**

Prognosis is better if respiratory status can be stabilized before treatment.

Reference

Wilson JM et al: Congenital diaphragmatic hernia–a tale of two cities: The Boston experience. J Pediatr Surg 1997;32:401.

Esophageal Atresia & Tracheoesophageal Fistula

- **Essentials of Diagnosis**
  - 85% have esophageal atresia with distal tracheoesophageal fistula (TEF), 5–7% pure esophageal atresia, 2–6% TEF alone; other configurations are rare
  - Symptoms and signs: asymptomatic in the first few hours of life; excessive drooling, choking, coughing; regurgitation, respiratory distress, cyanosis, scaphoid abdomen if pure esophageal atresia
  - Prenatal ultrasound shows polyhydramnios; chest and abdominal x-ray reveal blind esophageal pouch when nasogastric tube inserted
  - Workup: obtain chest and abdominal films with nasogastric tube; esophageal contrast study can verify fistula

- **Differential Diagnosis**
  - Rule out associated abnormalities (present in 50% of patients): vertebral, anorectal, cardiac, renal, radial limb

- **Treatment**
  - Decompressive gastrostomy if TEF is causing gastric distention; resection of fistula with primary repair of esophageal atresia
  - Indications: resolution or stabilization of pulmonary or cardiac abnormalities
  - Prognosis: 85–90% survival

- **Pearl**

Always evaluate for other congenital abnormalities.

Reference

Albanese CT et al: Pediatric surgery. In Way LW, Doherty GM (editors): Current Surgical Diagnosis & Treatment, 11th ed. McGraw-Hill, 2003.

Hirschsprung Disease

- **Essentials of Diagnosis**
  - Distal colon aganglionosis resulting in dysfunctional myenteric plexus; associated cardiac defects in 2–5%; trisomy 21 in 5–15%
  - Symptoms and signs include failure to pass meconium in first 24–48 hours of life, feeding intolerance, abdominal distention, bilious emesis, chronic constipation
  - Contrast enema shows transition zone distally
  - Workup: suction rectal biopsy is 85–90% sensitive

- **Differential Diagnosis**
  - Rectal or colonic atresia
  - Meconium plug syndrome, meconium ileus
  - Hypermagnesemia, hypocalcemia, hypokalemia
  - Hypothyroidism

- **Treatment**
  - Diverting colostomy for neonates with enterocolitis and Hirschsprung disease; Duhamel, Soave, or Swenson procedure at age 9–12 months or once proximal dilation has subsided after diverting colostomy
  - Prognosis: 80–90% maintain good bowel function

- **Pearl**

Bowel that looks abnormal on x-ray is the normal part; the normal-appearing distal segment lacks the ganglia.

Reference

Albanese CT et al: Pediatric surgery. In Way LW, Doherty GM (editors): Current Surgical Diagnosis & Treatment, 11th ed. McGraw-Hill, 2003.

Imperforate Anus

- ■ Essentials of Diagnosis
  - High imperforate anus: above the striated muscle complex or levator ani; absence of dimple or absence of gluteal fold
  - Low imperforate anus: rectal pouch descending into striated muscle complex; presence of anal membrane, dimple, or fold (usually); more favorable prognosis after reconstruction
  - 70% of cases associated with other abnormalities such as VACTERL: vertebral abnormalities, anal atresia, cardiac abnormalities, tracheoesophageal fistula and/or esophageal atresia, renal agenesis and dysplasia, limb defects
  - Symptoms and signs include distended abdomen, bilious emesis, irritability, failure to pass meconium
  - Workup: perform abdominal pelvic x-ray, pelvic ultrasound, voiding cystourethrogram, echocardiogram, spinal magnetic resonance imaging (MRI) or ultrasound, renal ultrasound, upper gastrointestinal (GI) study

- ■ Differential Diagnosis
  - Evaluate for VACTERL association: vertebral abnormalities, anal atresia, cardiac abnormalities, tracheoesophageal fistula and/or esophageal atresia, renal agenesis and dysplasia, limb defects

- ■ Treatment
  - High imperforate anus: diverting colostomy until at least 12 months of age, followed by (most commonly) posterior sagittal anorectoplasty and closure of rectourinary fistula
  - Low imperforate anus: cutback anoplasty (circumferential mobilization of anterior fistula and transposition to center of external anal sphincter)
  - Prognosis: approximately 20% mortality from other abnormalities

- ■ Pearl

Always evaluate for other congenital anomalies.

Reference

Albanese CT et al: Pediatric surgery. In Way LW, Doherty GM (editors): Current Surgical Diagnosis & Treatment, 11th ed. McGraw-Hill, 2003.

Intussusception, Pediatric

- ■ Essentials of Diagnosis
  - • 95% of cases are idiopathic; most commonly involve ileocecal valve; peak age is 6–9 months, but ranges from 3 months to 3 years
  - • Symptoms and signs include abdominal pain (colicky), vomiting, bloody stool, palpable mass in right abdomen (80–90% of cases)
  - • Contrast enema is 100% sensitive, showing lead point of intussusception, and is often therapeutic when performed under pressure

- ■ Differential Diagnosis
  - • Rule out peritonitis
  - • Consider possible lead-point abnormalities

- ■ Treatment
  - • Surgery: laparotomy and resection of intussusception if ischemic necrosis is present; laparoscopic reduction of intussusception if enema is unsuccessful
  - • Medications: contrast enema to reduce (60–80% successful); pneumatic preferred

- ■ Pearl

Excessively vigorous, successful reduction of necrotic intussusception is worse than leaving it in place for resection because it may allow peritoneal spillage.

Reference

Albanese CT et al: Pediatric surgery. In Way LW, Doherty GM (editors): Current Surgical Diagnosis & Treatment, 11th ed. McGraw-Hill, 2003.

Malrotation

- **Essentials of Diagnosis**
  - Varying degrees or absence of small bowel rotation; small intestine on the right and colon on the left with narrow superior mesenteric artery pedicle and Ladd bands lying across duodenum; 50–75% present in first month of life
  - Symptoms and signs include bilious emesis, abdominal distention, feeding intolerance, irritability
  - Upper GI series shows duodenojejunal junction to right of midline and some duodenal narrowing

- **Differential Diagnosis**
  - All other causes of childhood bowel obstruction

- **Treatment**
  - Ladd procedure
  - Resection of necrotic bowel
  - Appendectomy

- **Pearl**

Not all malrotation becomes symptomatic in childhood.

Reference

Albanese CT et al: Pediatric surgery. In Way LW, Doherty GM (editors): Current Surgical Diagnosis & Treatment, 11th ed. McGraw-Hill, 2003.

Necrotizing Enterocolitis

- **Essentials of Diagnosis**
  - Most frequent surgical condition in a neonate; associated with multiple comorbid conditions resulting in mucosal injury of the intestine
  - Symptoms and signs include abdominal distention; feeding intolerance; bilious emesis; occult or gross blood in stool; abdominal tenderness; abdominal wall edema, crepitus, or discoloration (suggest perforation); temperature instability; apnea; bradycardia

- **Differential Diagnosis**
  - Rule out perforation

- **Treatment**
  - Exploratory laparotomy if patient decompensates or does not improve after 24–72 hours of medical management; or if pneumoperitoneum, portal venous gas, abdominal wall erythema, or crepitus
  - Resection of necrotic bowel, proximal enterostomy, and distal mucous fistula
  - Medications: 90% can be managed with nasogastric tube decompression, bowel rest, broad-spectrum antibiotics, and correction of other comorbid conditions
  - Prognosis: mortality rate is 20–40%

- **Pearl**

  Prognosis is often dictated by the severity of associated illness.

Reference

Ladd AP et al: Long-term follow-up after bowel resection for necrotizing enterocolitis: Factors affecting outcome. J Pediatr Surg 1998;33:967.

Neuroblastoma

- ■ Essentials of Diagnosis
  - Most common extracranial solid tumor and most common abdominal solid malignancy of childhood
  - Associated with neurofibromatosis type 1, Beckwith-Wiedemann syndrome, Hirschsprung disease, musculoskeletal and cardiovascular malformations, Turner syndrome
  - Symptoms and signs include cervical mass, airway compression, abdominal mass, Horner syndrome, recurrent urinary tract infections, hydronephrosis
  - 24-hour urine collection shows elevated metanephrine, dopamine, and vanillylmandelic acid
  - CT or MRI demonstrates extent of disease and location of primary tumor, which can be found anywhere along the sympathetic chain

- ■ Differential Diagnosis
  - Wilms tumor
  - Any abdominal mass

- ■ Treatment
  - Surgery: resection of all gross tumor and regional nodes as well as vascular dissection
  - Medications: chemotherapy and radiation for high-risk tumors
  - Prognosis: 10–30% overall survival for high-risk tumors; 3-year survival of 40–97% (depending on stage)
  - Factors that place patients at high risk include age >1 year, stages III and IV, unfavorable Shimada classification (histology), N-*myc* amplification, no trk expression, 1p deletion, ferritin >142 ng/mL, lactate dehydrogenase >1500 IU/L

- ■ Pearl

Neuroblastoma may resolve spontaneously in young patients.

Reference

Shimada H et al: International neuroblastoma pathology classification for prognostic evaluation of patients with peripheral neuroblastic tumors: A report from the Children's Cancer Group. Cancer 2001;92:2452.

Pectus Excavatum/Carinatum

- **Essentials of Diagnosis**
  - Often is present at birth but becomes more pronounced as adolescence progresses
  - Symptoms and signs: excavatum causes posterior curve of sternum, with right side usually more curved; carinatum causes protruding sternum

- **Differential Diagnosis**
  - Underlying pulmonary dysfunction
  - Underlying cardiac dysfunction

- **Treatment**
  - Excavatum: osteotomy or Nuss bar placement in early or middle teenage years
  - Carinatum: osteotomy and sternal fracture
  - Surgery is indicated for severe deformity and psychosocial impact
  - Prognosis: recurrence rate is 5–15%

- **Pearl**

The psychosocial impact can be significant.

Reference

Nuss D et al: A 10-year review of a minimally invasive technique for the correction of pectus excavatum. J Pediatr Surg 1998;33:545.

Pediatric Abdominal Wall Defects

- **Essentials of Diagnosis**
  - Gastroschisis: associated with other abnormalities 10% of the time, most often intestinal atresia; associated with preterm birth
  - Omphalocele: associated with other abnormalities 50% of the time; nearly always occurs in full-term infants
  - Symptoms and signs: gastroschisis nearly always located to right of umbilicus, with inflamed bowel and foreshortened mesentery from exposure to amniotic fluid; umbilical cord is part of sac in omphalocele along with peritoneum
  - Prenatal ultrasound often shows the abdominal wall defect

- **Differential Diagnosis**
  - Associated congenital abnormalities
  - Intestinal atresia with gastroschisis

- **Treatment**
  - Primary surgical repair is possible in 60–70%; silicone rubber pouch or silo construction followed by gradual reefing and eventual closure
  - Giant omphaloceles: nonoperative initial therapy, gradual epithelialization, and closure months to years later
  - Complications: abdominal compartment syndrome, necrotizing enterocolitis (15% in gastroschisis), delayed ileus or intestinal dysmotility (especially in gastroschisis)

- **Pearl**

Always evaluate for other congenital anomalies.

Reference

Albanese CT et al: Pediatric surgery. In Way LW, Doherty GM (editors): Current Surgical Diagnosis & Treatment, 11th ed. McGraw-Hill, 2003.

Pediatric Airway Obstruction

- ■ Essentials of Diagnosis
  - Nasal causes include choanal atresia, teratoma, encephalocele
  - Oral-cavity causes include macroglossia, micrognathia, hypoplastic mandible with cleft palate
  - Pharyngeal and laryngeal causes include cysts or tumors
  - Acquired causes include foreign-body aspiration, acute epiglottitis
  - Symptoms and signs include restlessness, tachypnea, dyspnea, chest wall retractions, inspiratory stridor, respiratory arrest, drooling, dysphagia, fever (with epiglottitis)
  - Lateral cervical plain film shows edema of epiglottis and ballooning of pharynx; chest film shows aspirated foreign body
  - Perform lateral cervical film for suspected epiglottitis, laryngoscopy (in operating room under anesthesia) for suspected epiglottitis, bronchoscopy for aspirated foreign body

- ■ Differential Diagnosis
  - Rule out epiglottitis

- ■ Treatment
  - Surgery: tracheostomy for some obstructions; resection of tumors or cysts causing airway obstruction
  - Medications: third-generation cephalosporin for epiglottitis
  - Prevention: *Haemophilus influenzae* type B vaccine

- ■ Pearl
Always beware of epiglottitis.

Reference

Albanese CT et al: Pediatric surgery. In Way LW, Doherty GM (editors): Current Surgical Diagnosis & Treatment, 11th ed. McGraw-Hill, 2003.

Pediatric Intestinal Obstruction (Nonpyloric Stenosis)

- ■ Essentials of Diagnosis
  - Causes include intestinal atresia, intestinal duplication, mesenteric or omental cyst, Meckel diverticulum, foreign body, meconium ileus, annular pancreas
  - 10–20% of patients with abdominal wall defects have intestinal atresia
  - 90–95% of duodenal atresia is distal to ampulla; duodenal atresia associated with trisomy 21; cardiac anomalies
  - Symptoms and signs include bilious emesis, abdominal distention, irritability, maternal polyhydramnios, failure to pass meconium
  - Abdominal x-ray shows transition point of gas (intraluminal soap-bubble appearance in meconium ileus)
  - Workup: perform cystic fibrosis transmembrane regulator or sweat chloride test to document cystic fibrosis in patients with meconium ileus; echocardiogram in patients with duodenal atresia

- ■ Differential Diagnosis
  - Malrotation
  - Cystic fibrosis

- ■ Treatment
  - Primary anastomosis following short segmental resection; duodenoduodenostomy for annular pancreas and duodenal atresia
  - Operative retrieval of foreign body if symptomatic, if an alkaline battery, or if persists in 1 location for ≥1 week or stays several weeks in stomach
  - Prognosis: 93% 5-year survival after repair of intestinal atresia

- ■ Pearl

Always evaluate for associated anomalies.

Reference

Albanese CT et al: Pediatric surgery. In Way LW, Doherty GM (editors): Current Surgical Diagnosis & Treatment, 11th ed. McGraw-Hill, 2003.

Pediatric Neck Masses

- **Essentials of Diagnosis**
  - Causes include branchial cleft remnants, thyroglossal duct cysts, lymphadenopathy, vascular malformations and cystic hygroma, dermoid inclusion cysts, cervical thymic cysts
  - Branchial cleft remnants: usually present as cysts in late childhood, from angle of mandible (first cleft) down to lower third of sternocleidomastoid (second cleft); second-cleft remnants most common
  - Thyroglossal duct cyst: presents in late childhood as midline cystic neck mass, usually overlying hyoid
  - Suppurative lymphangitis: presents as painful, erythematous, draining mass
  - Hemangioma: becomes apparent after first few weeks of life, usually as blue, spongy, rubbery mass
  - Lymphangioma and cystic hygroma: typically present as asymptomatic masses

- **Differential Diagnosis**
  - Malignant lymph nodes
  - Infection with atypical bacteria, such as mycobacterium

- **Treatment**
  - Branchial cleft cyst: incision and drainage if infected; dissection and excision of cyst or fistula once infection resolves
  - Thyroglossal duct cyst: excision including mid point of hyoid and track up to base of foramen cecum
  - Lymphangioma or cystic hygroma: excision or sclerotherapy
  - Contraindications: do not perform excision in presence of active infection

- **Pearl**

Congenital lesions in the neck can present later in life.

Reference

Brown RL, Azizkhan RG: Pediatric head and neck lesions. Pediatr Clin North Am 1998;45:899.

Pediatric Thoracic Masses

- Essentials of Diagnosis
  - Resectable lung metastases: osteogenic sarcoma, soft-tissue sarcoma, Wilms tumor
  - Primary lung tumors: bronchial "adenoma" (malignant); bronchogenic carcinoma; pulmonary blastoma, sarcoma, inflammatory pseudotumor (benign); hamartoma (benign)
  - Mediastinal tumors: neurogenic; neurofibroma, lymphoma, teratoma
  - Symptoms and signs include cough with sputum, hemoptysis, chest pain, dyspnea, fever, postobstructive pneumonia
  - Chest CT can identify various causes of chest mass and relative locations; perform bronchoscopy for central lesions; thoracoscopy and possible biopsy for peripheral lesions

- Differential Diagnosis
  - All possible pediatric lung lesions

- Treatment
  - Formal resection (wedge or lobectomy) is indicated for nearly all pediatric thoracic masses
  - Excision of mediastinal lesions

- Pearl

Always control the primary tumor site before resection of pulmonary metastases.

Reference

Albanese CT et al: Pediatric surgery. In Way LW, Doherty GM (editors): Current Surgical Diagnosis & Treatment, 11th ed. McGraw-Hill, 2003.

Pyloric Stenosis

- **Essentials of Diagnosis**
  - Overall incidence is 0.1–0.4%; 7% incidence among children of affected parents; 4-fold higher incidence in males; higher incidence in first-born children
  - Symptoms and signs include nonbilious postprandial emesis at 2–12 weeks of life, becoming progressively projectile; palpable pylorus in right upper quadrant or epigastric region ("olive"); visible or palpable gastric peristaltic waves
  - Ultrasound shows hypertrophic pylorus (95% sensitive); upper GI study shows narrowed and elongated pylorus (95% sensitive)
  - Perform ultrasound of abdomen if diagnosis is in doubt; upper GI series if diagnosis still in doubt

- **Differential Diagnosis**
  - Overfeeding
  - Intracranial lesions
  - Pylorospasm; pyloric duplication
  - Antral web
  - Gastroesophageal reflux
  - Malrotation of the bowel
  - Adrenal insufficiency

- **Treatment**
  - Laparoscopic or open pyloromyotomy
  - Prognosis is excellent

- **Pearl**

Associated anomalies are rare.

Reference

Albanese CT et al: Pediatric surgery. In Way LW, Doherty GM (editors): Current Surgical Diagnosis & Treatment, 11th ed. McGraw-Hill, 2003.

Vascular Lesions, Congenital

- **Essentials of Diagnosis**
  - Arteriovenous malformation: uncommon, abnormal capillary formation during canalicular phase of development, mostly from pulmonary artery, rarely coronary artery
  - Vascular rings: abnormal development of aortic arches and branches with compression of trachea and esophagus; common complete rings: double aortic arch (67%), right aortic arch with left subclavian and ductus arteriosus (30%); incomplete rings: aberrant right subclavian originating from left side, and left pulmonary artery arising from right pulmonary artery
  - Symptoms and signs: arteriovenous malformation may be asymptomatic, otherwise dyspnea, congestive heart failure, angina; vascular rings cause symptoms of tracheal or esophageal compression or dysphagia lusoria (swallowing symptoms from anomalous right subclavian)
  - Imaging findings: for arteriovenous malformation, echocardiogram with Doppler is often diagnostic; for vascular rings, barium esophagram may be diagnostic; echocardiography can confirm diagnosis; occasionally angiography

- **Differential Diagnosis**
  - Tonsillitis
  - Esophageal mass
  - Mediastinal mass

- **Treatment**
  - Symptomatic vascular rings should be repaired; if double aortic arch, divide smaller of 2 arches; for complete rings, divide ligamentum arteriosum
  - Pulmonary artery slings: reimplantation of left pulmonary artery

- **Pearl**

Dysphagia lusoria is difficulty swallowing because of a right subclavian artery arising from the aortic arch, compressing the esophagus.

Reference

Van Son JA et al: Surgical treatment of vascular rings: The Mayor Clinic experience. Mayo Clin Proc 1993;68:1056.

Wilms Tumor

- **Essentials of Diagnosis**
  - Associated with Beckwith-Wiedemann syndrome, WAGR syndrome (Wilms tumor, aniridia, genitourinary abnormalities, mental retardation), neurofibromatosis, Denys-Drash syndrome, Perlman familial nephroblastomatosis
  - 1–2% incidence of bilateral disease; up to 7% multicentricity
  - Symptoms and signs include abdominal mass, pain, fever, hematuria
  - CT scan shows extent of disease in kidney and distant or nodal disease

- **Differential Diagnosis**
  - Neuroblastoma
  - Familial syndrome

- **Treatment**
  - Surgery: resection of tumor with inspection of contralateral kidney and sampling of regional nodes; resection is performed after chemotherapy or radiation therapy if bilateral disease (to spare renal function) or if major vessel involvement
  - Chemotherapy: vincristine and actinomycin D with doxorubicin added for stages III and IV
  - Radiation: for stage III, pulmonary or hepatic metastases, or all stages if unfavorable histology
  - Prognosis: 4-year survival is 78–97% (depending on stage)

- **Pearl**

Always evaluate for familial syndromes and bilateral disease.

Reference

Capra ML et al: Wilms' tumor: A 25-year review of the role of preoperative chemotherapy. J Pediatr Surg 1999;34:579.

Index